Research and Medical Practice:
their interaction

*The Ciba Foundation for the promotion of international cooperation in
medical and chemical research is a scientific and educational charity established by
CIBA Limited – now CIBA-GEIGY Limited – of Basle. The Foundation operates
independently in London under English trust law.*

*Ciba Foundation Symposia are published in collaboration with
Elsevier Scientific Publishing Company, Excerpta Medica, North-Holland Publishing Company,
in Amsterdam.*

Elsevier/Excerpta Medica/North-Holland, P.O. Box 211, Amsterdam

Symposium on

Research and Medical Practice: *London, 1976* their interaction

Ciba Foundation Symposium 44 (new series)

1976

Elsevier · Excerpta Medica · North-Holland
Amsterdam · Oxford · New York

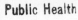

R
850
.S97
1976

☆

ISBN Excerpta Medica 90 219 4049 3
ISBN American Elsevier 0-444-15230-x

Published in July 1976 by Elsevier/Excerpta Medica/North-Holland, P.O. Box 221, Amsterdam and American Elsevier, 52 Vanderbilt Avenue, New York, N.Y. 10027.

Suggested series entry for library catalogues: Ciba Foundation Symposia.
Suggested publisher's entry for library catalogues: Elsevier/Excerpta Medica/North-Holland

Ciba Foundation Symposium 44 (new series)

Library of Congress Cataloging in Publication Data

Symposium on Research and Medical Practice, London, 1976.
    Research and medical practice.

    (Ciba Foundation symposium; 44 (new ser.))
    Bibliography: p.
    Includes indexes.
    1. Medical research--Congresses.   2. Medicine--Congresses.
I. Ciba Foundation. II. Title. III. Series: Ciba Foundation.
Symposium; new ser., 44.
[DNLM: 1. Research--Congresses.   2. Medicine--Congresses.
W3 C161F v. 44 1976/[W20.5 S984r 1976]]
R850.S95   1976   610'.72   76-24846
ISBN 0-444-15230-x (American Elsevier)

Printed in The Netherlands by Van Gorcum, Assen

Contents

Participants

Symposium on Research and Medical Practice held at the Ciba Foundation, London, 7–9 January 1976

SIR DOUGLAS BLACK (*Chairman*) Department of Health and Social Security, Alexander Fleming House, Elephant and Castle, London SE1 6BY, UK

*A. G. BEARN Department of Medicine, The New York Hospital-Cornell Medical Center, 525 East 68th Street, New York, NY 10021, USA

P. B. BEESON Veterans Administration Hospital, 4435 Beacon Avenue So, Seattle, Washington 98108, USA

R. W. BERLINER Yale University School of Medicine, 333 Cedar Street, New Haven, Connecticut 06510, USA

G. M. BULL MRC Clinical Research Centre, Watford Road, Harrow, Middlesex HA1 3UJ, UK

SIR ARNOLD BURGEN MRC National Institute for Medical Research, The Ridgeway, Mill Hill, London NW7 1AA, UK

E. J. M. CAMPBELL Department of Medicine, McMaster University, Hamilton, Ontario, Canada L8S 4J9

C. J. DICKINSON Department of Medicine, St Bartholomew's Hospital Medical College, West Smithfield, London EC1A 7 BE, UK

C. T. DOLLERY Department of Clinical Pharmacology, Royal Postgraduate Medical School, Hammersmith Hospital, Ducane Road, London W12 0HS, UK

---

* Contributed *in absentia*

A. C. DORNHORST   Medical Unit, St George's Hospital Medical School, Hyde Park Corner, London SW1X 7EZ, UK

L. EISENBERG   Department of Psychiatry, Harvard Medical School, Fegan 8, The Children's Hospital Medical Center, 300 Longwood Avenue, Boston, Massachusetts 02115, USA

T. M. FLIEDNER   Abteilung für Klinische Physiologie der Universität Ulm, Oberer Eselsberg M24, Niveau 3, D-7900 Ulm/Donau, West Germany

J. GELZER   CIBA-GEIGY Ltd, Pharma Research Department, CH-4002 Basle, Switzerland

H. H. HIATT   Harvard School of Public Health, 677 Huntington Avenue, Boston, Massachusetts 02115, USA

P. F. HJORT   Unit for Health Services Research, Institutt for Almenmedisin, Fr. Stangs gt 11–13, Oslo 2, Norway

R. LUFT   Department of Endocrinology and Metabolism, Karolinska Sjukhuset, S-104 01 Stockholm 60, Sweden

M. L. MARINKER   Department of Community Health, University of Leicester School of Medicine, 161 Welford Road, Leicester LE2 6BF, UK

P. MEYER   Physiologie-Pharmacologie, INSERM U 7, Hôpital Necker, 75015 Paris, France

S. G. OWEN   Medical Research Council, 20 Park Crescent, London W1N 4AL, UK

M. F. PERUTZ   MRC Laboratory of Molecular Biology, University Postgraduate Medical School, Hills Road, Cambridge CB2 2QH, UK

D. C. PHILLIPS   Department of Zoology, Laboratory of Molecular Biophysics, South Parks Road, Oxford OX1 3PS, UK

SIR GEORGE PICKERING   5 Horwood Close, Headington, Oxford OX3 7RF, UK

A. QUERIDO   Department of Clinical Endocrinology, Academisch Ziekenhuis, Rijnsburgerweg 10, Leiden, The Netherlands

P. J. RANDLE   Department of Clinical Biochemistry, University of Oxford, Radcliffe Infirmary, Oxford OX3 6HE, UK

SIR PHILIP ROGERS   Former Permanent Secretary, Department of Health & Social Security; Orchard House, 100 High Street, Wargrave-on-Thames, Berks RG10 8DE, UK

* R. SARACCI   Section of Epidemiology & Biostatistics, Laboratorio di Fisio-
logia Clinica CNR, via Savi 8, 56100 Pisa, Italy

SIR MICHAEL WOODRUFF   Department of Surgery, University Medical School,
University of Edinburgh, Teviot Place, Edinburgh EH8 9AG, UK

Editors: SIR GORDON WOLSTENHOLME (*Organizer*) and MAEVE O'CONNOR

* *Present address:* Unit of Epidemiology and Biostatistics, International Agency for Research
on Cancer, World Health Organization, 150 Cours Albert Thomas, 69008 Lyon, France

Introduction

Sir DOUGLAS BLACK

Department of Health and Social Security, London

In this opening section I shall only try to expand the title of the symposium, Research and Medical Practice. One theme we shall be discussing is: given that we can decide rationally on our objectives, what is the best process of making sure that the relevant research gets done? Sir Geoffrey Vickers, speaking about psychiatric research, once said:[1]

'Research workers are commonly regarded as geese who occasionally lay golden eggs. The three main ways of encouraging them to do so reflect different views of the extent to which this odd process can be either stimulated or directed.

'One way is to cosset any goose that actually has laid a golden egg, in the hope that it will lay some more. A second way is to specify the golden eggs required and offer rewards for them, hoping thus to move still unidentified geese to egg-laying. The third way is to go on increasing the goose farm in the hope that some statistical law will ensure that the number of golden eggs laid rises roughly in proportion to the number of birds capable of laying eggs at all'.

Vickers describes these as three alternative possibilities but I think that is a conceptual lapse: they are all possibilities which do not exclude the others.

Another theme we shall discuss concerns two caricatures of medical research. One is the ivory tower model, which can be summarized as 'knowledge for its own sake, regardless of cost and regardless of consequences'. The other caricature is of pure mission-oriented research, which stems from practical problems and is firmly prevented from deviating from them. Surely the truth, as so often, lies between the two extremes, and much of our time will probably be concerned with where the compromise lies between those two extreme views.

Scientists themselves must bear a good deal of responsibility for the confusion that surrounds the image of scientific research. We have both oversold this and undersold it from time to time. We have oversold it when we have been trying to arrange funds or even impress politicians. On the other hand we have often undersold it by shutting ourselves up in our ivory towers, and not deigning to explain the nature and purpose of our research activities.

Another type of problem is what I call the time-scale problem, which has again led to a certain lack of comprehension among lay people. Pressure groups or politicians expect instant answers to practically anything, whereas what I regard as the proper time-scale for solving those scientific problems that require major research is much longer, anything from three years to ten or twenty years. Interestingly, the time-scale of the scientist is much nearer that of the administrator than that of the politician, and I think this is one of the strengths of our society. A direct influence on policy by scientists is perhaps something that we dream of rather than something which will often be feasible in practice. As an ex-clinician I feel some sympathy with both those time-scales. In the ward or outpatient clinic one has to make a decision on a short time-scale, whereas in most investigative work one has to try to come to a decent decision by taking time over an accumulation of planned observations.

We begin our meeting with what might be called main-line clinical research on the 'seats of disease', the syndromes of dysfunction, and on clinical phenomenology, before we get to treatment, and all the dilemmas this brings. After that we reach problem-solving in science—something in which we might all have an interest—and the detection of relevance in the more basic types of research. Health service considerations come next, and finally we shall hear about the role of government in the control of medical research, and about biomedical research on the international scene.

Reference

[1] VICKERS, G. (1968) The promotion of psychiatric research. *British Journal of Psychiatry* *114*, 925–934

Delineation of clinical conditions: conceptual models of 'physical' and 'mental' disorders

LEON EISENBERG

Department of Psychiatry, Harvard Medical School, and Children's Hospital Medical Center, Boston, Massachusetts

Abstract The dysfunctional consequences of the Cartesian dichotomy have been enhanced by the power of biomedical technology. Technical virtuosity reifies the mechanical model and widens the gap between what patients seek and doctors provide.

Patients suffer 'illnesses'; doctors diagnose and treat 'diseases'. *Illnesses* are experiences of discontinuities in states of being and perceived role performances. *Diseases*, in the scientific paradigm of modern medicine, are abnormalities in the function and/or structure of body organs and systems. Traditional healers also redefine illness as disease: because they share symbols and metaphors consonant with lay beliefs, their healing rituals are more responsive to the psychosocial context of illness.

Psychiatric disorders offer an illuminating perspective on the basic medical dilemma. The paradigms for psychiatric practice include multiple and ostensibly contradictory models: organic, psychodynamic, behavioural and social. This mélange of concepts stems from the fact that the fundamental manifestations of psychosis are disordered behaviours. The psychotic patient remains a person; his self-concept and relationships with others are central to the therapeutic encounter, whatever pharmacological adjuncts are employed.

The same truths hold for all patients. The social matrix determines when and how the patient seeks what kind of help, his 'compliance' with the recommended regimen and, to a significant extent, the functional outcome. When physicians dismiss illness because ascertainable 'disease' is absent, they fail to meet their socially assigned responsibility. It is essential to reintegrate 'scientific' and 'social' concepts of disease and illness as a basis for a functional system of medical research and care.

In the Gospel according to St Matthew,[1] Jesus eluded the efforts of the Pharisees and the Herodians to lure him into treason by his cautious injunction: 'Render therefore unto Caesar the things that are Caesar's and to God the things that are God's.'[1] Similarly, the Cartesian dichotomy between matter and soul[2] can be viewed as a device that, since it surrendered a domain the church

3

claimed for itself, served to disengage biology from the church. The several Gospel accounts[1,3,4] agree that the Pharisees 'took counsel how to entangle him in his talk' 'so as to deliver him up to the authority and jurisdiction of the governor' but that Jesus was 'aware of their malice'; 'marvelling at his answer, they were silent' 'and went away'. Descartes on the other hand developed his philosophic dualism in order to reconcile his devout Catholicism with his mechanistic view of physiology rather than in an effort to avoid Galileo's fate. Whatever the original motives behind the two ways of partitioning the world, their adoption can be viewed as a pragmatic, time-buying stratagem for diminishing the threat to established authority, in the one instance secular, in the other theological. These concordats have been honoured in the breach as well as in the observance. Nonetheless, both have constrained the subsequent development of powerful social institutions.

As has so often happened in the history of ideas, what was at its inception liberating became in time restricting. The Cartesian disjunction freed biology (and thence medicine) to turn its full powers to the elucidation of physiological and pathological mechanisms in an epoch when natural science was able to develop methods and concepts for investigating only such matters. Yet the very success of the enterprise, most particularly in the past half century, has caused soul or mind to recede so far into the background of contemporary medical thought as to yield so narrow a perspective on problems of patient care as to seriously hamper the physician's efforts to provide that care. I refer here not so much to the insufficient attention given to psychiatry within the medical curriculum, although that is not an unimportant problem, as to the altogether inappropriate conceptualizations of illness provided for the student in his or her medical education. In the United States, this view was crystallized in the Flexner report,[5] a document which set the conditions for both the flowering of what is best in American medicine and the proliferation of the difficulties that now beset it on every side. The prodigious accomplishments of the new biology, institutionalized as the fundamental science to be applied in medical practice, further reified the Cartesian mechanical model. Working models of the disease process determine the data that physicians gather, inform the ways in which 'facts' are integrated into a diagnosis, and circumscribe the boundaries of interventions designated as therapeutic. The momentum of the technological imperative to do what we have the virtuosity to do (without pausing to consider whether it is worth doing) drives the physician's hand and brings him increasingly into conflict with what the patient seeks from him. Moreover, what has been called the new morbidity—with functional disorders and chronic illness displacing acute infections as the predominant challenges to the medical care system—is not only unresponsive to technology, but is in significant ways worsened by it. The ability to salvage congenital anomalies and to prolong vegetative existence with cardiopulmonary bypass machines and other devices raises questions of meaning and quality in life which strip away the illusion that technology is value-free.[6]

To sharpen discussion, I will set forth a somewhat overstated contrast between lay and professional perspectives without attempting to provide fully comprehensive and logically exclusive definitions.[7] What matters for the purposes of our symposium is the headlines, rather than the fine print, if we are to confront the major conceptual barriers to a responsive health care system.

To state it flatly, patients suffer 'illnesses'; physicians diagnose and treat 'diseases'. Let me make clear the distinction I intend: illnesses are *experiences* of discontinuities in states of being and in social role performance; diseases, in the scientific paradigm of modern medicine, are *abnormalities* in the *structure* and *function* of body organs and systems. I will employ this semantic distinction in the discussion that follows, though I acknowledge that illness and disease are synonymous in contemporary English usage.

Illness and disease, so defined, do not stand in a one-to-one relationship. When disease is extreme, as in diabetic ketoacidosis or in the terminal stages of malignancy, its pervasiveness makes illness inevitable. However, disease may occur in the absence of illness: the person with hypertension may be asymptomatic and therefore unconcerned when the physician who measures his blood pressure becomes alarmed; he may stop taking the prescribed medication because it makes him 'ill', even though he is told it will mitigate his 'disease'. Only when the hypertension leads to congestive failure or hemiplegia will the person become a patient and agree with his doctor that he is sick; even then the agreement may be limited to a common perception that a *problem* exists which each is likely to formulate in quite different terms.

Similar degrees of organ pathology may generate quite different reports of distress, differences determined by culture, expectation and setting. Zola[8] has described strikingly different complaint patterns in Italian and Irish patients with 'objectively' similar medical conditions. Beecher[9] has noted the greater reliance on morphine analgesia among civilian accident victims than among military battle casualties with comparable traumatic injuries. Calin and Fries,[10] in a systematic follow-up of 'healthy' blood donors positive for the histocompatibility antigen HLA-W-27 (an antigen previously identified as a marker for ankylosing spondylitis), found that about one-third of these ambulatory and undiagnosed individuals had symptoms of inflammatory disease and X-ray findings pathognomonic for the clinical entity. Here we confront the variability not only of disease expression in a genetically susceptible population but also of the medical index of suspicion for its diagnosis in the face of the ubiquity of chronic low back pain (also present in 10% of the control donors without W-27 who were simultaneously surveyed).

These few examples must suffice to illustrate the variability of the experience of illness in the presence of ascertainable disease of comparable severity. The other side of the coin is the problem of illness in the absence of detectable organ pathology, for which conversion hysteria provides a convenient paradigm. Its recognition is as ancient as Egyptian medicine (19th century B.C.); the term we still employ stems from Greek medicine (5th century B.C.). The regnant theories of its cause have changed from wandering of the uterus through demoniacal possession to psychological determination.[11] More importantly, its prevalence and its phenomenology have changed *pari passu* with the changes in ideas about it.[12] Rather than reviewing this historical evolution in detail, let us take a moment to consider the patients so meticulously studied by Charcot at the Salpêtrière.[13] Whatever his patients' initial complaints, by the time they had been shown repeatedly to the attentive medical audiences who flocked to his celebrated lectures, they came almost uniformly to exhibit all four phases of Charcot's 'major hysteric crisis' in the course of their medical acculturation. This presents, in microcosm, a culture-bound syndrome emerging from the interaction between the professor and his clientele.[14] Let it be clear: the patients were ill before they saw Charcot; what changed was the patterning of the symptoms; in a way, doctor and patient shared a *folie-à-deux*. He expected what they produced; they came to produce what he expected. It was the evolution of the clinical syndrome that had been altered, not its initiating pathogenesis. That had anteceded his intervention; yet his ideas, as they interacted with lay belief systems, in turn became part of the common culture. With culture change, the flamboyant manifestations of hysteria have diminished sharply in frequency.[12] Epidemics[15,16] in susceptible, usually rural, populations are still occasionally reported. The less dramatic and more diffuse psychosomatic syndromes have not only replaced the anaesthesias and paralyses of yesteryear as culturally constructed and legitimated responses to life stress but have also come to constitute a major fraction of medical practice.[17]

The shifting pattern of symptoms among military neuropsychiatric casualties provides another illustration of the shaping of the response to stress by culture which channels overt expression into explicit syndromes of illness. What DaCosta had described as 'irritable heart' or 'neurocirculatory asthenia' among soldiers in the American Civil War had been reified as 'disordered action of the heart' by British physicians at the time of the First World War. By the Second World War, cardiac symptoms, though still prominent, were less exclusive; the congeries of symptoms were reformulated in such diagnostic categories as 'battle fatigue' or 'combat neurosis'. Concomitantly, conversion symptoms (blindness and paralysis) were less often encountered in the Second than the First World War.[18]

The point of interest here is not the terminology but the changes in the observed manifestations, in which other symptoms had displaced the cardiac ones from the centre of medical attention. Indeed, in the Second World War, military psychiatrists noted the local character of prevalent clinical syndromes; that is, there were differences in the patterns observed at different fronts. More-over, the course of illness was observed to alter as the mode of management was changed. Prompt treatment near the front and rapid redeployment resulted in far less chronicity than when neuropsychiatric casualties were shipped back to distant hospitals.[19] What remains enigmatic is the relationship between official military figures and the actual prevalence of casualties. Factors like unit morale, effective leadership and specific battle conditions, as well as modes of management, influence incidence as well as course. To an unknown extent, we face a problem in classification; that is, the same constellation of signs and symptoms can be ascribed to medical causes (for example, cardiac malfunction), they can be regarded as instances of cowardice, or they can be labelled combat neurosis. It is also likely that actual rates of casualty are a function of the behavioural options which shared belief makes available to the community. Now that neurasthenia, a concept from Western medicine widely adopted in China and Taiwan (A. M. Kleinman, personal communication), is no longer an officially tenable diagnosis in the People's Republic of China, it would be most instructive to know what—if any—syndrome of illness has replaced it as a mode of response to stress.

If conversion hysteria serves as a convenient example of 'illness without disease', it also provides an apparent contradiction to the thesis that, for contemporary medicine, disease is organ pathology. Hysteria is to be found in the official medical classifications of 'disease'. In part, its tenure is a heritage of the past when it was the province of neurology; in part, it may be supposed by some to yield its secrets one day to more sophisticated biomedical research into its pathogenesis. However, it is precisely hysteria as a prototype of the 'myth of mental illness' that has been singled out by proponents of labelling theory[20] for use when they criticize physicians for 'medicalizing deviance'. Moreover, for many physicians, the so-called functional disorders represent problems of uncertain legitimacy and continuing debate over such concepts as malingering or secondary gain (misuse of the sick role, in sociological termin-ology).

My argument thus far has stressed the discrepancy between disease as it is conceptualized by the physician and illness as it is experienced by the patient.

To that I have added an emphasis on the way the patterning of illness is influenced by medical concepts as they permeate the general culture—which is something that has, of course, always been the case. Practitioners of the healing arts have existed for as long as professional functions have been specialized in human society. In a recent excavation of a Neanderthal burial site, a skeleton some 60000 years old was found close to pollen grains from eight flower species, seven of which are still extant and known for their medicinal properties.[21] This unlikely botanical clustering suggests bouquets purposefully gathered and laid down at the interment of a medicine man or shaman.

Whether or not healers appeared on the scene quite so long ago, medical lore is integral to every existing human culture.[22] With the historical evolution of a people, the healer, initially a repository of folk tradition, becomes highly specialized. He is 'called' to his role by personal experiences or attributes that set him off from others; he may be apprenticed to older practitioners and undergo a period of intensive preparation; he acquires arcane knowledge and the gift of communicating with the gods and spirits. Because he must expose himself to, and overcome, the dark forces that produce illness, he is deemed to possess great powers. The principal social functions of the medicine man reside in his ability to diagnose, to prescribe ritual actions designed to overcome illness, to cast a prognosis, and to legitimate the mysteries of death.[23] He names and explains just as we name and explain, though he and we employ very different explanatory systems. All belief systems (and we must acknowledge that this includes our own) are culture-bound. They make little sense out of context despite their persuasiveness to those brought up to share the same frame of reference. They change as the society which generates them changes—and as specialization of professional function permits the development of bodies of learned knowledge. To the extent that these new conceptions become common property, they may displace, merge with or simply coexist by the side of older lay beliefs, despite what appear to be logical incompatibilities. In developing countries, patients quite regularly employ the services of health practitioners of widely different persuasions, sometimes consecutively and sometimes simultaneously, as if to leave no source of relief untapped. Within such a society, as one moves from the low, usually preliterate healing tradition through the 'high' tradition (formal, scholarly and élite) and finally to imported western medicine, one observes widening gaps in shared belief, in social class and in effective communication between patient and practitioner.[24] This is more readily recognized in an exotic context; that is, when it occurs in another country. We ignore, at peril to our understanding, the extent to which British and American patients seek out marginal practitioners[25] and obtain as much (or as little) relief as orthodoxy is able to provide for such chronic disorders as low back pain.[26] What besets the western physician is a difference in degree and not in kind from what troubled his predecessors.

However, the very limitations of their technology kept indigenous healers more responsive to the extra-biological aspects of illness, for it was chiefly those aspects they could manipulate. Our success in dealing with certain disease problems breeds the ideological error that a technical fix is the potential solution to all. It would be absurd to suggest that we should forego the power of western medicine in deference to shamanism. It is essential to enquire how we can expand our horizons to incorporate an understanding of illness as a psychological event. Indeed, our worship of restricted and incomplete disease models can be viewed as a kind of ritual or magical practice in itself.

To what extent can we anticipate help from psychiatry in resolving these dilemmas? Of necessity, psychiatry has retained a greater concern than other fields of medicine for subjectivity and social context; the reasons are intrinsic to the specialty. The inherent nature of its clinical problems centre on distress and disturbed behaviour; other practitioners refer to it patients with ailments that stubbornly refuse to respond to conventional biomedical measures and patients whose behaviour is viewed as problematic for the health care system; the disorders it treats are peculiarly sensitive to psychosocial interventions; the epidemiology of psychiatric problems strongly implicates social influences as concomitant if not causal variables. Yet I must acknowledge at the outset that psychiatric theories reflect the conceptual confusion that afflicts the rest of medicine. If I venture to sketch their main outlines, it is because psychiatry has available to it a more catholic if incomplete and inconsistent set of concepts. In this sense, it may provide fruitful leads for a more comprehensive theory of medicine.

In what follows, I will focus on the psychoses. They provide the most convenient bridge to other medical disorders, in that the disease–illness dichotomy remains a central preoccupation. The concepts of the psychotic process that provide the paradigms for psychiatric practice include multiple and manifestly contradictory models:[27] the organic or *medical* model—genetically based aberrations in biogenic amine metabolism; the *psychodynamic*— developmental and experiential in origin; the *behavioural*—maintained by environmental contingencies; and the *social*—disorders of role performance. This potpourri of doctrines stems from the fact that psychosis manifests itself in disordered behaviour. With full recognition of its physiological roots, behaviour is simultaneously a function of developmental history and interpersonal context.

The medical model of psychosis is as ancient as the monograph 'On the Sacred Disease' attributed to the Hippocratic corpus. It affirms 'And men ought to know that from the brain and the brain alone arise our pleasures, joys, laughter and jests, as well as our sorrows, pains, griefs and tears... By the same organ we become mad and delirious, and fears and terrors assail us... and dreams and untimely wanderings... All these things we endure from the brain, when it is not healthy...'.[28] This view reached its apogee in the 19th century with neuropathology triumphantly 'explaining' general paresis. When the confident expectation that other psychiatric disorders would reveal themselves under the microscope failed to be fulfilled, the disease model was supported by only a hardy few, to be revivified within the past two decades by the discovery of psychotropic drugs, new evidence for genetic diatheses, and neurochemical findings. Those psychiatrists who follow the medical model pay close attention to signs and symptoms as the foundation of differential diagnosis because it is the identification of the clinical entity that enables the doctor to predict the expected course and to determine the appropriate treatment. Drugs and electric shock, measures directed at the somatic matrix, are the keys to management; psychosocial measures are adjunctive. Both implicitly, by the medical character of the treatment given, as well as explicitly, in the explanatory models provided, the patient is led to believe that he has a disease, similar to other diseases, for which he need feel no culpability. A good patient, however, is expected to follow the medical regimen. The diagnosis legitimates the sick role but simultaneously confers responsibility for compliance.

The psychiatrist in the psychodynamic mode views psychosis as the end-result of the vicissitudes of pathological life experience; that is, of arrested development, distortions in reality perception, impaired adaptive responses. Syndrome diagnosis is almost irrelevant to treatment because its fundamental method is one of uncovering the idiosyncratic past and facilitating its re-integration into new patterns of meaning. The patient's aberrations stem from acting towards persons in his current environment as though they were the important figures from his past. Thus, exploring the relationship between doctor and patient underlies the therapeutic process of correcting interpersonal distortions. In contrast to the conventional medical model of disease and treatment, the patient is enjoined to play a central role in his own rehabilitation. Although he is acknowledged as sick, he holds veto power over his recovery. The very terms employed—flight into illness, resistance, secondary gain, degree of motivation—imply his participation in his illness. The developmental emphasis implicates his family, as does the inclusion of family members in group and family psychotherapy. If the psychodynamic model preserves the dignity of the patient as a free person, it exacts a price in the responsibility it confers on patient and family for causing or contributing to the sickness.

The behavioural model evolved from the application of operant conditioning theory, a contribution from academic psychology, to the management of clinical problems. In this paradigm, abnormal behaviour is learned behaviour; by definition, it persists because other people in the patient's environment unwittingly maintain that behaviour by rewarding him for exhibiting it and by ignoring or punishing him when he deviates from it. There is no 'disease' to be identified and treated; rather there is a constellation of behaviours that require to be changed. What matters are the relationships between output and input: the black box between is not an important focus of interest; subjective self-report is an unreliable guide to its contents and the details of its wiring are indifferent to the output/input analysis. The equivalent of diagnosis is the task of identifying the rewards that have maintained undesirable behaviours. Treatment consists of the design of a contingency response programme in which rewards are delivered only for those constructive behaviours whose frequency is to be increased. So long as total control can be maintained over the responsive environment, what the patient thinks is a matter of indifference; it is what he does that counts. And that can be externally controlled, at least so long as others cooperate. The recent extension of the behavioural model to biofeedback methods[29] provides a powerful technology with which physiological as well as behavioural functions can be modified. Non-manipulable motivational elements do, of course, enter the scene with voluntary patients who must contract to adhere to the programme. But the behaviourist's client, primarily a responder rather than an initiator, is analogous to the medical patient who is expected to follow doctor's orders. This is, at first glance, a curious coincidence; the behavioural technician specifically disclaims interest in the internal workings of the machine, whereas these are focal concerns for the biomedical technologist; however, the identical outcome in the structure of the therapist–client relationship stems from the shared premise that the forces producing illness exist in spheres apart from the patient as a thinking and feeling person.

The fourth model, the social, emphasizes the individual's role in the social system. It is the character of his interrelations with the persons who make up his life space, and that of the social role to which he is assigned that constitute the source of his disorder. In this context, emphasis is placed on the effect of a psychiatric label as a powerful mechanism which casts the individual in the role of patient and generates a set of expectations he is coerced into filling. This proposition is particularly difficult for physicians to accept; it makes them into society's gate-keepers and jailers,[30] in complete contravention of the profession's self-image of its function as beneficent healer. Yet there are facts that cannot be swept away. When Pinel in France and Tuke in England at the end of the 18th century introduced the moral treatment of the insane, they were considered radicals for striking the chains from the 'violent' insane. Contrary to the conventional wisdom, the violence of patients diminished rather than increased once the restraints were removed. The restraints themselves had generated much of the resistance which was the ostensible justification for their use. The importation of moral treatment to American shores was criticized on the ground that American patients were inherently in need of greater restraint because American society was more anarchic; yet the results of humane care on overt behaviour of patients were similar to those in Europe. A more recent example of the pervasive influence of the social field on behaviour is the identification of the social breakdown syndrome[31]—a behaviour pattern that characterizes the neglected chronic schizophrenic patient. Superimposed on the initial psychosis is the deadly levelling effect of the institution as a total society. The observed pattern of behaviour results not from the 'disease' but from the experience of anonymity and alienation and the assignment to the role of chronic patient. Contrariwise, the devolution of the state hospital system in the United States began before the massive use of psychotropic drugs; the change resulted from reorganization of the system, altered admission and discharge policies, and the development of community services. The drugs were, however, instrumental in accelerating and sustaining that process.[32] In its most extreme form, the sociological model places the principal determinants of behaviour entirely in the social field and leaves little or no room for biological and psychological factors 'internal' to the patient. To epitomize by analogy, human behaviour in a dynamic social field may be likened to the movements of iron filings in a changing magnetic field.

How are we to reconcile these models? Each captures important facets of clinical reality, yet disregards or even denies others. We lack the equivalent of Lorentz transformation equations that would enable us to move from one inertial frame of reference to another. A comprehensive and inclusive general theory of disease–illness would subsume the relations that hold true within particular coordinate systems and specify the limiting conditions. That theory has yet to be written; even then it will be no more than a provisional guide for comprehending the clinical world.

Models are ways of constructing reality, ways of imposing meaning on the chaos of the phenomenal world. This is not to deny the independent reality of that world but to emphasize that it does not present itself to us organized in the ways we come to view it. The models physicians use have decisive effects on medical behaviour. The models determine what kind of data will be gathered; phenomena become 'data' precisely because of their relevance to a particular set of questions (out of the possible sets of questions) which is being asked. Once in place, models act to generate their own verification by excluding phenomena outside the frame of reference the user employs. Models are indispensable but hazardous because they can be mistaken for reality itself rather than as but one way of organizing that reality.

Error is compounded when abstractions are reified and diseases are regarded as things. Virchow[33] wrote: 'Diseases are neither self-subsistent, circumscribed, autonomous organisms, nor entities which have forced their way into the body, nor parasites rooted on it but... represent only the course of physiological phenomena under altered conditions'. Even within the definition of disease as organ pathology, disease is not an entity but a relational concept. From this vantage point, Engelhardt[34] has brought the central issue into focus: 'If disease is viewed as a relation, one can then choose those aspects of the relation most easily manipulable; that is, most easily treated... Theory thus becomes an instrument of action: one chooses a theory to highlight variables open to easy influence'.

In his actual practice, the physician employs what Polanyi[35] terms 'personal knowledge'; that is, he combines 'tacit' models of illness with more or less explicit models of disease. If they were to be spelt out and deliberately set side by side, these tacit and explicit concepts would display logical incompatibilities. That they are held simultaneously indicates that clinicians mediate between medical models of disease and popular models of illness just as do the patients who employ concurrently the services of herbalists, shamans and doctors. The resolution of the tensions between contradictory models occurs in practical action. Health practitioners behave differently from what they say they do when they are asked to describe their actions.[24] Closer attention to 'tacit' knowledge should enable us to construct more comprehensive clinical models of disease–illness.

My argument for the necessity of a more universal perspective on illness is not an academic exercise in the philosophy of medicine. What we think affects what we do. Biomedical concepts have yielded major dividends for certain classes of disease problems. However, they are not only irrelevant to others, but misleading because they misdirect our efforts. The image of the doctor as technician contributes to the paradox of patients being dissatisfied at a time when the profession considers that its powers are at their greatest. We generate false expectations for cure that lead to malpractice suits when medical fallibility rather than personal incompetence is the issue. Virtuosity in performing too readily becomes an end in itself and blunts sensitivity to purpose. As Burge and his associates[36] noted in a recent article on the treatment of acute myeloid leukaemia 'The present preoccupation with intensive therapy appears to blind physicians to the poor quality of life which their patients lead. The aim of treatment is too often to induce a haematological remission (an irrelevance to the patient) rather than to improve the quality of life'. The modern doctor's dilemma is a product of our new biological powers. Only when it is possible to delay death does it become meaningful to ask whether it should be delayed. That question did not have to be asked when the best we could do was to diminish suffering, now as then a value most would agree upon.

From the time of the first healers, patients came to them to seek relief from discomfort and dysfunction. They found what they sought and they honoured the provider. Symptom relief under medical care is the commonest outcome for most episodes of illness. Historically, this bonus to medicine as craft has been a plague to medicine as science. The benefits patients obtained have been attributed to the procedures in fashion rather than to the social dynamics of the medical encounter. With the growth of experimental sophistication in clinical trials, such benefits have been labelled 'placebo' effects: that is, sources of variance that complicate experimental design. 'Placebo' has become almost an epithet suggesting charlatanism rather than a marker for an extraordinary and quite fundamental characteristic of good medical care. Of course, we need controls in clinical trials if we are to evaluate new remedies. But we ought equally to seek an understanding of our therapeutic heritage rather than disdaining it, as the 'hard' scientist does, or being deceived by it, as many practitioners are.

Curt dismissal of 'placebo effects' is symptomatic of the widespread contempt in which psychotherapy is held—as though it were ineffective because no one brand has been shown to be clearly superior. What has hounded research in this area has been the effectiveness of psychotherapeutic methods in abating symptoms. When two-thirds of a comparison group reports itself improved, a new mode of treatment will need remarkable powers indeed to generate a significant difference.[37] More appropriate is a reversal of the traditional paradigm (the search for differences) so that just those common attributes which underlie the generally good symptomatic outcomes can be identified. It is only when changes in social effectiveness (in contrast to changes in symptom scores) are examined that it becomes possible to demonstrate gains from psychotherapy over and above those resulting from medication.[38]

The therapeutic benefit derived from the medical presence, I contend, is evidence for the mediating role of psychosocial factors in the genesis and maintenance, as well as repair, of the experience of illness. In a given case, these factors may hold the centre of the stage or be peripheral to the main drama. They are never absent in the ill person until consciousness lapses; even then, they continue to operate in the responses of family and community. For most of their history, healing theory and practice have responded to psychosocial factors in symbolic and tacit ways; what is called for now is systematic social and behavioural research in medicine, supported by resources comparable in magnitude to those we have so profitably devoted to the biomedical enterprise. There can be no pretence that the psychosocial field yet possesses methods of like investigative elegance and power. Equally, there need be no reason to doubt our ability to fashion such methods once we acknowledge how crucial they are to understanding contemporary health problems.

Medical care is a complex social process, embedded in the cultural matrix and laden with values. Critics warn us of the hazards of technical iatrogenesis;[39] let us be similarly alert to the potential for psychosocial toxicity.[40] Symptom relief can be purchased at too heavy a price; not only may the identification of a malignant process be delayed but both doctor and patient may become captives of a misleading mystique. The outcomes that matter are long-range as well as episodic. Is the patient wiser after the transaction: that is, more proficient at self-care or more dependent on the doctor as anodyne? Both modern and traditional medicine share that hazard. If cure is in part a function of belief, how shall we prepare the practitioner for conveying confidence while retaining the private scepticism necessary for an investigative attitude?

Problems of ethics abound. We cannot deliberately fabricate belief systems and practices for experimental study. It is precisely here, however, that research into cross-cultural medicine may prove particularly illuminating.[23] We can take advantage of 'natural' cultural variation to compare and contrast outcomes. The chastening discovery that other theories of disease, and practices based on them, can produce benefit helps to free us from medical ethnocentrism.[6] Once illness is reconceptualized as a disruption in an ongoing biosocial matrix, we will be less likely to pursue disease as a thing-in-itself. The chase after that will o' the wisp recalls a remark attributed to Gertrude Stein. Commenting on a nondescript American town, she said 'When you get there, you discover there's no there there!'

ACKNOWLEDGEMENTS

I acknowledge with special thanks the stimulating discussion and criticism provided by my colleague, Professor Arthur M. Kleinman, now of the University of Washington, Seattle, in the preparation of this paper. The work discussed was supported, in part, by a grant from the Robert Wood Johnson Foundation to study the physician-patient relationship in cross-cultural perspective.

Discussion

Black: Your distinction between 'disease' and 'illness' reminds me that in the days when antihypertensive drugs had even more side-effects than they have now, a patient being treated with ganglion-blocking drugs said to me 'When I feel well I am ill and when I feel ill I am well'.

Your four models or paradigms for psychiatric practice lead me to question the application of the term 'relevant research'. Obviously, whether research is relevant depends on which model is being used, and in particular on whether the right model is picked for a particular patient. Who do you think should choose the model: the physician or the patient?

Eisenberg: Psychiatric exclusivism (total adherence to a single model) regrettably still exists but, happily, is on the wane. To the extent that it persists, it puts a burden on the general practitioner to match his patient's needs to a particular psychiatrist's therapeutic model. Far better would be sufficient eclecticism among my colleagues for them to choose the treatment model most appropriate to the salient features in a given case. We would still face the problem of mismatch between doctor's and patient's view.

In clinical practice it is striking how often there is failure of understanding between patient and physician. The patient comes in with his own notion of his experience and his own theories to explain it. The physician usually doesn't even bother to ask. Yet if one understands the 'theory' on which the patient is acting one can avoid certain errors in prescribing practice. Some of the things that follow logically enough from medical theory are totally irrelevant to the patient's beliefs, especially a patient from a different culture.

Woodruff: A person with some behavioural aberration due to organic disease, for example a frontal lobe tumour or hyperparathyroidism, will receive very different treatment according to whether he is examined by a psychiatrist or a neurologist. Surely there is a great danger in over-specialization or attachment exclusively to one model or a restricted number of models?

Eisenberg: Exactly. There are disasters on both sides. The physician's specialty rather than the presenting problem often determines the course of investigation and treatment. If you have a tension headache and go to a neurologist you may end up undergoing examination by angiography or pneumoencephalography; if you have a brain tumour and go to a psychiatrist, then heaven help you!

Bull: Should you separate those four models quite so firmly? For example, if thiourea, which has a bitter taste, was used as an operant conditioner, obviously some of the population would respond and some would not—some communities may like a bitter taste anyway and a different sort of conditioning would be produced.

Eisenberg: There is no disagreement between us. The dilemma is that those who are committed to a model offer it as a comprehensive explanation of all behaviour. My contention would be that each model is in itself insufficient to explain behaviour fully. In fact, they overlap; phenomena are multiply determined and they interact. The social critics of psychiatry do not believe that psychiatric disorders exist apart from the labels that 'create' them. I have no sympathy with that view. Behavioural disorders are known to every society by indigenous standards and most can be recognized cross-culturally. But when our critics force us to acknowledge that some modes of 'treatment' superimpose social disabilities on top of the primary deviation, I think they are absolutely correct. My objection is that social labelling theory, which is a powerful theory, is proposed *in place of* disease theory, and I cannot accept that. Physicians, on the other hand, sometimes take the view that if they can't see illness under the microscope, there is nothing there.

Campbell: You have told us that in some cultures people who feel ill go to different sorts of practitioners. A number of these patients would probably like to have some structure, some frame of reference, to explain what is happening to them. Do they go to different people for different treatments for what they think is the same thing, or do they think they have different things causing the same illness?

Eisenberg: There are pragmatic levels at which individuals choose appropriate practitioners. For example, in Nigeria an individual with a broken bone will go to a bone setter, not to a shaman. If he has an illness that we would call psychosomatic, he may go to a shaman. If he has a condition that is clearly recognized as responding to antibiotics, he treks as far as he must to go to a hospital and get a western doctor. People are rather good at that. In Taiwan, for a number of functional complaints, patients may consult several different classes of practitioners during the *same* episode of illness. For illiterate patients, the lowest level (least formally educated) practitioner is the one whose beliefs are most consonant with their own and with whom they have the closest understanding. But they also respect alternative modes. Herbalists differ from the shamans, who go into a trance during which they answer questions about illness as the vehicle for the voice of the god. In Taiwan, one remarkable system makes use of ancient Chinese characters painted on tiles hanging on a wall in the temple. After the patient has thrown dice to determine the appropriate fate, the interpreter (the Tang-ki) uses the designated character to give the prognosis for the illness. The patient is unable to read the characters himself or herself. According to traditional accounts, these characters are simply 'read' much as a scholar would read an ancient language. However when my colleague, Dr Arthur Kleinman, spoke to the Tang-kis and watched their interactions with the patients, he found that they were quite discriminating in the way they interpreted the characters. That is, if the literal prognosis was bad and it looked as if the patient couldn't take the news, the interpreter changed the 'reading' to suit his assessment of the patient's needs. They were pragmatic psychotherapists in their own special way.

Kleinman visited patients who went to several categories of healers, that is to priests, shamans, physicians trained in Chinese medicine, and western-trained Chinese physicians. His work (in progress; not yet published) notes an inverse correlation between the degree of training of the physician and the amount of functional relief obtained by the patient. The western-trained Chinese doctor was so remote from his lower-class patients that he was not at all responsive. (I should point out that Dr Kleinman was not studying acute medical or surgical illness but the run of the mill complaints brought to the office.)

Campbell: Do the patients go to the lowest-level person, acquire a model from him and then go to the higher level people for more effective treatment for that model, or do they accept a confusing mix of models?

Eisenberg: They accept a confusing mix of models. That is the striking thing about it.

Meyer: Is there much difference between the attitude in Taiwan and that in Europe? In Europe many people see, one after another, a university doctor, a private practitioner, and eventually a charlatan or quack of some kind. This attitude of consulting several doctors at the same time is perhaps just a sign of anxiety.

Black: Whether it expresses anxiety or not, I am sure that seeing a number of doctors produces anxiety.

Eisenberg: One might look at it quite the other way round. When families in Cleveland were asked to keep diaries of their experience of illness, it was found that only about a quarter of illness episodes got as far as the doctor's office.[41] People consult the neighbourhood druggist, their next-door neighbours, their wives or mothers – mothers make a lot of health decisions within the family. There are varying beliefs about what constitutes an illness serious enough to go to a healer, whether a pharmacist or physician. It seems to me that we shall fall far short in our conceptualization of health care, and in training physicians to provide health care, if we don't begin with the whole range of things that are done before the patient comes to the doctor and with what the patient thinks about that medical transaction. Complaints about the doctor not listening are among the major sources of dissatisfaction in outpatient care.[42] Certainly within the last ten years studies have revealed huge gaps in compliance with medical regimens.[43] Not long ago *The Lancet* published a letter describing an elderly man who had been regularly visiting the outpatient department of a large hospital in London and who had responded to none of the many drugs that were prescribed. He was finally admitted to hospital and the home visitor who went to his flat found intact and untaken, a dozen different medications prescribed in the previous months. Doctors have not taken into account this whole aspect of the patient as a behaving person in a family setting and with his own ideas about what is happening.

Saracci: You said that all belief systems, including that on which present-day scientific medicine is based, are culture-bound. But not all belief systems are equally well equipped conceptually to become conscious of being culture-bound. To be conceptually equipped for something is not the same as actually being ready for it: all processes pushing towards self-consciousness in fact meet strong resistance, whatever the belief system within which they take place. Still, the key advantage of the scientific belief system is that it is more conceptually prepared to become conscious of its structure and character than other systems are of theirs.

Eisenberg: The fact that our scientific system is conscious of itself as a system is certainly one of the distinctions between magical 'pre-scientific' thinking and what we believe, but we have underestimated the amount of logical and scientific understanding that pre-literate peoples have. We have been guilty of believing that science is so rational that new facts always persuade us to abandon old theories. But scientists are reluctant to give up theories. Kuhn has pointed out that it takes more than just additional facts to force a new paradigm on us.[44] It is not a matter of abandoning the methods of science but of insisting that scientific methods be extended beyond research in cellular pathology to the analysis of psychological and social interactions as determinants of illness.

Burgen: You mentioned shamans and shamanism in primitive societies. What about the residue of shamanism and its inheritance in our own society, in other words the priestly role?

Eisenberg: Physicians as 'shamans' have been essential to society since its beginnings. We should not give up the shamanistic role without examining its consequences. I am distressed by the extent to which some people in the USA argue that the courts and the law can better resolve problems that in the past were left to doctors and their patients. I say this in full awareness that physicians are far from perfect. Some are stupid and some are arrogant; yet in the aggregate all the small errors they make may be outweighed by the benefits in individual problem-solving that are possible if certain decisions are left in the traditional medical sphere. Leaving decisions there may be preferable to trying to settle in the law courts such problems as when brain death has occurred and when life support can be withdrawn (as in the Quinlan case). What is needed is more attention to these issues in the training of physicians, who should understand better what responsibility they bear. That is, they should understand that they can bring a great deal of comfort to the dying patient and the patient's family: they should not withdraw from the family on the ground that a doctor's job is to cure and that if he can't do that, he has no further role. Healing has been respected by mankind for many thousands of years and it is only recently that we have acquired powerful agents that make a decisive pharmacological or surgical difference; the shamanistic role can bring much relief to people. I am always astonished at how little of what we do in general medical practice has other than a shamanistic function. When I stress that 'placebo' ought to be an honourable rather than a dishonourable term, that is the point I want to make.

Burgen: In your account of Taiwan, you emphasized the number of practitioners whom the patient consulted. In our western society we tend to have one practitioner, a physician, whom we consult. However well trained that physician is, however multifunctional, however sympathetic to the social setting, do you expect one person to carry out those multiple functions as effectively as several people?

Eisenberg: That is a profound and difficult question to answer. In the States, we seem to be riding off in all directions at the same time. That is, we are training nurse-practitioners or physician's assistants, and at the same time we are proposing to train primary physicians with less emphasis on biomedical science. Soon there will be no difference between these categories of health workers. If a doctor is to be a biological technician who deals with the difficult clinical problems in a tertiary-care hospital, we will be training a very different kind of physician. Can one person embody all these skills? Does scientific training, by restricting what is 'interesting' to the doctor, make him technically incapable of meeting psychological needs? I don't know if that is true. If one becomes intrigued by problems of organic pathophysiology, can one also be intrigued by human qualities, by personal interaction with the individual patient? With embarrassment, I remember my own behaviour as an intern, spending half an evening in the emergency room trying to keep an old man with a stroke out of our hospital because we expected another patient with multiple myeloma in the morning; we were doing a study of that disease, which seemed much more interesting than a stroke. Something had gone seriously wrong with me and that system when I behaved that way.

Querido: In our society, in contrast to developing countries, the scientific approach to problems has taken up a large section of our way of looking at reality. I suppose that it is only possible to say that a person has an illness, and not a disease, if one has first excluded the presence of disease. But in practice diagnosing a disease is much simpler than *excluding* the presence of a disease. What is the practical solution? I certainly agree with you that illness needs multiple treatment and help.

Eisenberg: The problem of 'excluding' disease is one of the central issues in the orientation of medicine towards public health issues. Some years ago a study of general practitioners gave a rather low rating of their calibre.[45] They didn't always do all the things that hospital specialists thought essential. It seems to me that one has to train medical students that a pragmatic and probabilistic approach is essential. The first time the patient shows up with a headache the probability that he has a brain tumour is very small. If every initial headache is examined for a brain tumour, the number of people injured by radiation and diagnostic procedures will far exceed the number who will be saved by early identification of a tumour. The basic problem in educating the physician is to look at the probabilistic decision-making table that he has to follow. He has to consider the risks of the procedures that he undertakes on behalf of the patient. The disease has to be fairly likely before he goes far in investigating it by diagnostic procedures that carry risk of injury. We sometimes make our students so eager to identify the esoteric and unusual diagnosis that the patient is put at risk rather than being helped.

Hjort: The basic nature of man is such that he cannot face ambiguities over a long time. Therefore he cannot face four models: he needs one. Our biomedical model is in the process of being overtaken by less credited models. Unless we modify and improve our model, we will suddenly discover that it has been discarded by the public. Therefore, we should make a better model, rather than settle for four separate ones.

Marinker: There is confusion between technology and science in the way in which we train doctors to look at problems. I think it was Sir Peter Medawar who said that a physician's work consists of making imaginative conjectures and then validating them. But the clinical method we teach the student is not the one the physician uses. The physician doesn't use a screening procedure for each patient he sees but makes first an imaginative conjecture about the patient's headache or cough. That is the essence of the scientific method, whether it concerns the discovery of the configuration of the DNA molecule or the elucidation of the cause of a cough or sore throat. One of the things that has gone wrong with medical education is that we teach doctors that some kind of inductive process like a screening procedure is necessary before a problem can be elucidated.

Eisenberg: Obviously there is not a single way of teaching, and the stereotypes of failures that I offered appear in some settings but not others. The success of biomedical science is extraordinary. Since I left medical school, the number of agents that produce powerful effects in contrast to the number with which medicine was previously equipped has grown to an extraordinary extent. However, from public health statistics, overall life expectancy doesn't seem to have been much affected by those agents. Social factors seem to have been of much more consequence. The reasons patients come to doctors have to do with much more than disease in the narrow sense. Here, where we are looking at what research can contribute to medical practice and how one might design research strategy, we must also ask what makes people behave as patients, and why they come to surgeries. If we simply place more and more reliance on molecular biology *alone*, we are doomed to be unable to meet the needs of patients. If we knew more about what makes people come to doctors and then designed a system that included physicians, physicians' assistants and other forms of personnel, we might begin to come into some reasonable relationship to the demand. In a country like the USA, which is now spending $ 118 thousand million for a grossly inadequate health care system, we can't just provide more of the same: it has to be something different.

References

1 MATTHEW 22: 15-21
2 DESCARTES, R. (1649) The passions of the soul, in *Philosophical Works of Descartes*, vol. 1, pp. 345-348 (translated by E. S. Haldane & G. R. T. Ross, 1951), Dover, New York
3 MARK 12: 13-17
4 LUKE 20: 19-26
5 FLEXNER, A. (1910) *Medical Education in the United States and Canada*, The Carnegie Foundation for the Advancement of Education, Bulletin No. 4, New York
6 EISENBERG, L. (1975) The ethics of intervention: acting amidst ambiguity. *J. Child Psychology and Psychiatry and Allied Disciplines 16*, 93-104
7 FABREGA, H. (1972) Concepts of disease: logical features and social implications. *Perspectives in Biology and Medicine 15*, 583-616
8 ZOLA, I. K. (1966) Culture and symptoms: an analysis of patients' presenting complaints. *American Sociological Review 31*, 615-630
9 BEECHER, H. K. (1956) Relationship of significance of wound to the pain experienced. *Journal of the American Medical Association 161*, 1609-1613
10 CALIN, A. & FRIES, J. F. (1975) Striking prevalence of ankylosing spondylitis in 'healthy' W-27 positive males and females. *New England Journal of Medicine 293*, 835-839
11 VEITH, I. (1965) *Hysteria: The History of a Disease*, University of Chicago Press, Chicago
12 CHODOFF, P. (1954) A reexamination of some aspects of conversion hysteria. *Psychiatry 17*, 75-81
13 GUILLAIN, G. (1959) *J.-M. Charcot: His Life – His Work* (translated by P. Bailey), Hoeber, New York
14 MUNTHE, A. (1930) *The Story of San Michele*, Dutton, New York
15 SMITH, H. C. T. & EASTHAM, E. J. (1973) Outbreak of abdominal pain. *Lancet 2*, 956-958
16 SIROIS, F. (1973) Les épidémies d'hystérie: revue de la littérature. *L'Union Médicale du Canada 102*, 1906-1915
17 STOECKLE, J., ZOLA, I. K. & DAVIDSON, G. (1964) The quantity and significance of psychological distress in medical patients. *Journal of Chronic Diseases 17*, 959-970
18 BAKER, S. L. (1975) in *Comprehensive Textbook of Psychiatry/II* (Freedman, A. M., Kaplan, H. I. and Sadock, B. J., eds.), pp. 2355-2367, William & Wilkins, Baltimore
19 Medical Department, U.S. Army (1974) *Neuropsychiatry in World War II*, Vol. 2, U.S. Government Printing Office, Washington, D.C.

20 SZASZ, T. (1964) *The Myth of Mental Illness*, Hoeber/Harper & Row, New York
21 SOLECKI, R. S. (1975) Shanidar IV, a Neanderthal flower burial in Northern Iraq. *Science (Washington, D.C.) 190*, 880-881
22 LESLIE, C. (ed.) (1976) *Toward a Comparative Study of Asian Medical Systems*, University of California Press, Berkeley
23 KLEINMAN, A. M. (1974) The cognitive structure of traditional medical systems. *Ethnomedicine 3*, 27-45
24 KLEINMAN, A. M. (1975) Explanatory models in health care relationships, in *Proceedings of the 1974 International Health Conference on Health of the Family*, pp. 159-172, National Council for International Health, Washington, D.C.
25 FIRMAN, G. J. & GOLDSTEIN, M. S. (1975) The future of chiropractic: a psychosocial view. *New England Journal of Medicine 293*, 639-642
26 KANE, R. L., LEYMASTER, C., OLSEN, D. *et al.* (1974) Manipulating the patient: a comparison of the effectiveness of physician and chiropractic care. *Lancet 1*, 1333-1336
27 LAZARE, A. (1973) Hidden conceptual models in clinical psychiatry. *New England Journal of Medicine 288*, 345-351
28 *Hippocrates: The Genuine Works*. Translated by Francis Adams (1886) Vol. 2, p. 344, William Wood, New York
29 MILLER, N. E. (1969) Learning of visceral and glandular responses. *Science (Washington, D.C.) 163*, 434-445
30 ZOLA, I. K. (1972) Medicine as an institution of social control. *Sociological Review 20*, 487-504
31 GRUENBERG, E. (1967) The social breakdown syndrome: some origins. *American Journal of Psychiatry 123*, 1481-1489
32 EISENBERG, L. (1973) The future of psychiatry. *Lancet 2*, 1371-1375
33 VIRCHOW, R. (1958) *Disease, Life and Man*, Stanford University Press, Stanford, California
34 ENGELHARDT, H. T. (1974) Explanatory models in medicine: facts, theories and values. *Texas Reports on Biology and Medicine 32*, 225-239
35 POLANYI, M. & PROSCH, H. (1975) *Meaning*, pp. 22-45, University of Chicago Press, Chicago
36 BURGE, P. S., RICHARDS, J. D. M., THOMPSON, D. S. *et al.* (1975) Quality and quantity of survival in acute myeloid leukemia. *Lancet, 2*, 621-624
37 LUBORSKY, L., SINGER, B. & LUBORSKY, L. (1975) Comparative studies of psychotherapies: is it true that 'everyone has won and all must have prizes'? *Archives of General Psychiatry 32*, 995-1008
38 WEISSMAN, M. M., KLERMAN, G. L., PRUSSOFF, B. A. *et al.* (1974) Treatment effects on the social adjustment of depressed out-patients. *Archives of General Psychiatry 30*, 771-778
39 ILLICH, I. (1975) *Medical Nemesis: The Expropriation of Health*, Calder & Boyars, London
40 FOX, R. C. (1976) The medicalization and demedicalization of American society. *Daedalus*, in press
41 DINGLE, J. H., BADGER, G. F. & JORDAN, W. S. (1964) *Illness in the Home*, Western Reserve Press, Cleveland, Ohio
42 READER, G., PRATT, L. & MUDD, M. (1957) What patients expect from their doctors. *Modern Hospital 89*, 88-94
43 HAGGERTY, R. J. & ROGHMANN, K. J. (1972) Non-compliance and self-medication. *Pediatric Clinics of North America 19*, 101-115
44 KUHN, T. S. (1970) *The Structure of Scientific Revolutions*, 2nd edn., University of Chicago Press, Chicago
45 PETERSON, O. L. (1956) *An Analytical Study of North Carolina General Practice 1953-1954*, Association of American Medical Colleges, Evanston, Ill.

Structural determinants of disease and their contribution to clinical and scientific progress*

ALEXANDER G. BEARN

Department of Medicine, New York Hospital–Cornell Medical Center, New York

Abstract The recognition of structural correlates with disease provided a release from the Hippocratic humors which dominated the approach to medicine for more than a thousand years. During recent decades an increasingly reductionist approach to structure has enabled such correlations to extend from those easily visible to the naked eye to those whose resolution requires sophisticated electron microscopy. Although recognition of clinical–pathological correlations has evident advantages, there are instances, such as diabetes mellitus, where such recognition appeared to lull investigators into believing that the pathogenic mechanisms underlying the disease had been found. Moreover, the recognition of a structural abnormality, such as the extra chromosome in Down syndrome, may sometimes have delayed rather than accelerated research on metabolic aspects of the disease. The advances in medical understanding that have proceeded from a correlation of structure with function have enabled diseases to be investigated at different levels. This has led to a more sophisticated redefinition of the meaning of clinical–pathological correlations and to the surprising finding that immense structural variability can be tolerated by the human organism without its function being recognizably perturbed. Indeed, some molecular variations of structure lead to a distinct biological advantage under singular environmental conditions. Finally, where molecular structure is known in its most intimate detail, the distinction between structure and function becomes less easy to discern.

Conventional wisdom, precariously based on historical precedent, has led us to consider clinical–pathological correlations as well-defined, clinically recognizable entities associated with a distinct morphological variation in an organ. One of the first, apparently clean-cut, clinical–pathological correlations was described by Richard Bright in 1827, when he observed a positive correlation between an abnormal-looking kidney and patients dying from diseases 'which terminated in dropsical effusion'. But Bright was notably cautious in his

---

* Dr Bearn was unable to attend the symposium and this paper was presented on his behalf by Sir Gordon Wolstenholme.

interpretation, for, having observed the altered appearance of the kidneys, he says 'whether they are to be considered as the cause of the dropsical effusion or some other disease, cannot be unimportant'. With enviable crispness he concludes, 'If it were possible to arrive at a perfect solution of these questions we might hope to obtain the highest reward which can repay to our labors, an increased knowledge of the nature of the disease and improvement in the means of its treatment'.[1]

But before I update this theme and focus on current medical and biological approaches to the structure–function relationship, it is worth emphasizing that it was the recognition of structural correlates with disease processes which provided a happy though long-delayed release from the metaphysical world of Hippocratic humors that had dominated and shackled the scientific approach to medicine for more than a thousand years. With the publication of *De Sedibus* by Morgagni in 1761,[2] the importance of the relationship of structure to function first became recognized, and since then this concept has increasingly contributed to medical progress. The mere collection of facts, however—the witless assembly of ill-defined diseases and symptoms, divorced from any pathological correlation—frequently delayed the advance of medical knowledge. A veritable lepidopterists' paradise was erected by Boissier de Sauvages, who in 1768, in his *Nosologia Methodica*, grouped diseases into ten classes, 295 genera, and 2400 species.[3]

Although a mere recitation of the advances in medical knowledge that have flowed from Morgagni's initial observations would be both self-evident and repetitious, I would be remiss if I did not refer to Bichât, who in 1800 was the first to point out that pathological changes occurred not so much in organs as in tissues. These observations led directly to the classic work of Virchow, who, in his turn, transferred the seat of disease from the tissues to individual cells, and in so doing introduced the enduring concept of cellular pathology.[4]

I would like to focus here on the value of considering structural and functional correlations in medicine today. I shall restrict myself to developing five major interrelated themes:

(1) That ascribing a causal relationship to a correlation between a pathological observation and a clinical syndrome is an inductive quicksand and scientifically perilous: for such uncritical acceptance may not only delay our biological understanding but also delude us into the belief that effective therapy is close at hand, and that additional efforts directed towards the fundamental understanding of the biological process are an unnecessary luxury.

(2) That the relationship between the structural anomaly and a clinical entity has, on occasion, had the undesirable effect of decreasing research on basic

mechanisms when, in fact, the structural relationship delineated should have been used to refocus and redirect the question posed.

(3) That immense structural variability can be tolerated by the human organism without biological or clinical function being recognizably perturbed.

(4) That recognition of functional variation and clinical disease should allow structural variation to be predicted and should encourage its recognition, just as structural observations can lead to previously unrecognized function being demonstrated.

(5) That when molecular structure is known in its most intimate detail, the distinction between structure and function becomes less easy to discern, and when structure and function finally merge they should be distinguished only when operationally expedient to do so. Indeed emphasis in future should be focused on pathogenesis of disease rather than on structure–function relationships.

First, to exemplify the importance of recognizing clinical–pathological correlations, and at the same time to illustrate the dangers of over-interpreting such correlations, I shall sketch the evolution of our knowledge of diabetes mellitus.

The story begins in 1889 in the laboratory of the medical clinic in Strassburg, where von Mering and Minkowski showed that diabetes mellitus followed surgical extirpation of the pancreas. 'After complete removal of the organ, the dogs became diabetic. It has not to do with a transient glycosuria, but a genuine lasting diabetes mellitus, which in every respect corresponds to the most severe form of the disease. The appearance of such disease comes without exception, unless the animals have died from the immediate effects of the operation'.[5] The clinical–pathological correlation moved to a finer hierarchical level when, in 1900, Opie described hyaline degeneration of the pancreatic islands of Langerhans in diabetes.[6] The advance of the correlation to a cellular level led Sharpey-Schafer to postulate in 1916[7] that diabetes is due to the lack of a hypothetical internal secretion—a prediction, if you will, of a functional correlate of the structural abnormality. This prediction was fulfilled in 1922 when Banting and Best showed that the 'intravenous injection of an extract from the dog's pancreas, removed from seven to ten weeks after ligation of the ducts, invariably exercises a reducing influence upon the percentage sugar of the blood and the amount of sugar in the urine'. Soon afterwards it was shown that the administration of insulin could be life-saving to diabetic patients and thus the problem of a disease commonly lethal in early adult life appeared to have been solved in a mere thirty years.

The glib belief that since diabetes is a disease of insulin deficiency, it could be rapidly and effectively 'cured' by the administration of insulin is, however, a myth, as we have painfully learned. Today, some fifty-five years later, the disease seems more enigmatic and more obscure than in 1922. It is perhaps not generally appreciated that in the United States diabetes, or at least the recognition of the disease, has increased about 300% over the last fifteen years. It is the second leading cause of blindness, and the third cause of death. In 1950 there were 1.2 million diabetics in the United States; the estimation now is that there are over ten million, yet the population has increased by only 50%.

Insulin is localized in the granules of the β cells of the pancreas; it stimulates cellular uptake of glucose and aids in the conversion of glucose to glycogen in both liver and muscle. It does, of course, a great deal more: it stimulates cellular uptake of amino acids and thus stimulates protein synthesis; it also stimulates nucleotide uptake into DNA and RNA. Lipids are not ignored, for insulin stimulates lipogenesis. The picture became more complicated when glucagon, another hormone affecting carbohydrate metabolism, was found by de Duve and his colleagues to be present in the α cells of the pancreas.[9] Indeed, as is now well known, many diabetics have insulin antibodies and are not insulin-deficient, a view which could not be substantiated until methods of measuring insulin in the blood had been developed.

For many years, the cellular mechanisms which underlay the endocrinological effects of insulin remained obscure. It appears that insulin is non-covalently bound to specific cell receptors and then becomes biologically active. The exact mechanism of the functional triggering which follows insulin binding is still unknown. When the receptor molecule is bound by insulin, production of cyclic AMP is blocked and its level falls. Insulin may have a direct physiological effect on cyclic AMP, or the binding of insulin may affect the conformation of the cell and modulate enzymic processes indirectly. Interestingly, there appear to be additional insulin-binding sites on the cell which can be uncovered by treatment with phospholipase. Even though it is not known how insulin action is modulated, it is possible that in some patients insulin resistance may be related to the number of binding sites on the cell; alternatively the binding sites may be blocked by insulin antibody.[10, 11] The mouse with recessively inherited diabetes has a reduced number of insulin-binding sites. Could the obese insulin–resistant form of diabetes be caused by homozygosity for a specific gene at a single locus, which decreases the number of insulin receptor sites or affects insulin binding? Whether there are fewer insulin-binding sites in the very rare recessively inherited form of diabetes which occurs in childhood and is invariably associated with blindness is at present unknown.[12] The enzyme glucagon also binds specific receptor sites on cell surfaces; adenylcyclase is then promptly activated and this effect is probably related to the functional activity of glucagon. Clearly our understanding of the pathogenesis of diabetes has reached a different level of cellular understanding in recent years and is now intimately associated with the pathobiology of membrane function.

That genetic influences play a role in the aetiology of diabetes has long been known[13,14], though their precise role has been difficult to identify. This field is moving rapidly after years of being in the doldrums. The juvenile form of diabetes appears to be linked to the *HLA* locus, which raises the possibility that certain individuals possessing a particular *HLA* type may be prone to develop the disease. Recent studies suggest, but by no means prove, that individuals who possess *HLA* 8 and *W* 15 alleles are about twice as likely to get juvenile diabetes as those who have other alleles, whereas the probability that maturity-onset diabetes will develop is independent of the specific alleles at the histo-compatibility locus.[15] Although more studies are needed before too much significance is attributed to these findings, they raise the possibility that pancreatic damage by specific viruses may be important in the aetiology of juvenile diabetes in man. In certain strains of mice encephalomyocarditis virus (M variant) replicates exclusively in the pancreas and causes diabetes. At various times, mumps, Coxsackie B3 and B4 antibodies have been claimed to exist in high concentration in patients with juvenile diabetes, but the evidence is still inconclusive. In contrast, there is no evidence of a specific *HLA* prevalence in maturity-onset diabetics, and the role of viruses in the aetiology of this form of diabetes is less persuasive.[16]

The recent observation[17] that there is an increase in the basement membrane glycoproteins in diabetes, coupled with the finding that in diabetic mice, as well as in patients with diabetes, 6–10% of the haemoglobin is in the glycosylated form (haemoglobin A_{1c}) underlines the difficulties in unravelling the complexities of the disease.

The story of diabetes mellitus illustrates the way in which clinical–pathological correlations, structure–function relations, have illuminated our understanding of the disease. It also illustrates how easy it is to misinterpret such correlations. We have today an abundance of hints and encouraging observations extending to clinical pathology, endocrinology, cell surfaces and specific binding sites, antibodies, genetic susceptibility, and viral infections. The frequency of the disease or diseases—for it would clearly be folly to regard diabetes as a simple entity—appears to be steadily increasing, or at least increasingly recognized. Therapy is still inadequate except in the short term, and the efficacy of insulin and tight control of the disease in preventing the vascular complications is highly questionable. Indeed, the end of the story that seemed so elegantly solved in 1922 is not yet in sight.

I would like to turn now to another example in which the clear recognition of a structural correlate, although its contribution to our understanding of the disease was profound, appeared to lessen interest in the understanding of disease at the molecular level.

Before Lejeune and his colleagues observed in 1959[18] that mongolism, now more gracefully termed Down syndrome, was associated with trisomy 21, the only biological correlation of consequence was the information, painstakingly obtained by Penrose, that there is a striking increase in the frequency of the disease among children of elderly mothers. By using Fisher's method of partial correlation coefficients, Penrose was also able to show that the age of the father is quite immaterial.[19]

Before Lejeune's observations there was a plethora of papers on the supposed biochemical basis of mongolism. At various times proteins, carbohydrates, vitamins and phospholipids were blamed for the clinical manifestations. Most of the experiments reported were poorly conceived, methodologically rocky, statistically naive, and spectacularly inconclusive.[20] Nevertheless, interest in the biochemical basis of the disease was present. With the recognition that trisomy 21 was regularly associated with mongolism, that interest wafted away. The cause of mongolism was now known—it was trisomy 21. But the problem of causation had *not* been resolved; this new knowledge merely enabled the question to be rephrased. In what way does the extra chromosomal material with its accompanying genetic information exert its physiological effects? Three specific genes are now known to be located on chromosome 21 (the genes for ribosomal RNA, antiviral protein and superoxide dismutase 1) (V. A. McKusick, personal communication), but their significance in the aetiology of the disease is far from clear. Certainly the simplistic belief that the presence of three chromosomes meant that there would be a 50% increase in the product of any gene located thereon was quickly shown to be false.[21] I mention this example to show the ease with which a clinical–pathological correlation appeared to have blunted biochemical interest. The finding of trisomy 21 may not have made the pathogenic biochemical quest any easier, but it certainly did not make it less worth while.

Indeed, as recently as 1975, an entire volume was published in which more than fifty syndromes, loosely described as malformation syndromes, were associated with additions, subtractions and rearrangements of structurally identifiable chromosomes.[22] In the flurry of syndrome collecting (and I in no way wish to make this sound belittling), there is a notable absence of concern about how the observed chromosomal oddities achieve their functional effects, and indeed whether they all result in recognizable biological effects. However, renewed interest has emerged and doubtless the field will move again in a more sophisticated and focused direction.[23] The molecular mechanisms responsible for the functional abnormalities associated with chromosomal aberrations form a rapidly moving field of investigation. The initial structure–function relationship of trisomy 21 and Down syndrome was a spectacular finding, but it is only the beginning of our understanding of the disease.

The third point I want to raise concerns the immense structural variation which can be tolerated by the human organism without any functional effect becoming obvious. E. B. Ford defined genetic polymorphism as 'the occurrence together in the same locality of two or more discontinuous forms of a species in such proportions that the rarest of them cannot be maintained merely by recurrent mutation'.[24] It is one of the most commonly observed and least understood phenomena in biology. Polymorphism cannot be maintained at conventional mutation rates if the variants number more than 1% of the total. Allison's observation that the sickle cell gene conferred an advantage on those exposed to malaria and thus accounted for the high gene frequency[25] was received with such enthusiasm that there was a Gadarene rush to explain all balanced polymorphisms in an analogous fashion. Even here our physiological understanding of the structure–function relationship may be subtly changing. Erythrocytes that lack the Duffy group are resistant to simian malaria (*Plasmodium knowlesi*), and many people in West Africa, where vivax malaria is rare, lack the Duffy blood group. Perhaps the Fy^a or Fy^b blood groups are receptors for vivax.[25] Except for malaria, the reasons why balanced polymorphisms exist are scarcely known, and this has led to the current debate on whether there are neutral mutations, a subject which cannot be developed here. But whether these variations are advantageous or have been so in the distant past, begs the question: they certainly exist. A number of years ago we became interested in the iron-binding protein in serum transferrin—at least a dozen electrophoretically different transferrins have now been shown to exist, yet so far no obvious advantage or disadvantage can be observed.[27] Harris and his colleagues have suggested that in normal man, as in drosophila, between 24 and 40% of the loci controlling the synthesis of soluble proteins and enzymes are electrophoretically polymorphic.[13]

Although not all structural variations can be detected electrophoretically it can be calculated that perhaps 16% of gene loci coding for enzyme structure are heterozygous. Thus an immense, totally unpredictable, variation in the structure of proteins can occur with no detectable functional consequence.

Chromosomal polymorphism also exists in man to an extraordinary extent and appears not to be associated with overt functional change. This field, too, is moving rapidly and influencing our traditional concepts of the structure–function relationship.

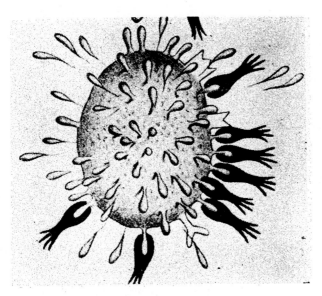

Fig. 1. Ehrlich's concept of cellular antigen receptors (from Ehrlich 1900).

Fourthly, there are many instances in biology and medicine of a structura variation of a particular type being predicted from purely functional consider- ations. To begin with an early example, Harvey in *De Motu Cordis* asserted that if his view of the circulation was correct then small vessels must exist to connect the arteries to veins.[28] In 1661 Malpighi described in compelling detail those very structures which Harvey had predicted must exist on functional grounds—the capillaries.[29]

In 1900, Ehrlich made the explicit prediction that the cells of the body must have receptors for foreign antigens (Fig. 1).[30] It is curiously ironic that although he was so immersed in haematology he never suspected that the cell he was postulating was the lymphocyte. Generations of investigators specializing in work on the lymphocyte took little notice of Ehrlich's suggestion. Seventy-five years later, it seems that many of the world's best immunological laboratories are studying and dissecting in intimate detail the receptors for antigens on T and B type lymphocytes.[31]

As a result, we now know that in the syndrome of chronic lymphatic leukae- mia B cells alone proliferate, whereas in acute leukaemia there is a mixture of pure B cells and pure T cells. Another example where structural variation has led to the recognition of a new function comes from so-called hairy-cell leukae- mia. The morphological characterization of leukaemic cells by the light micro- scope has been known for decades, yet recently, with the scanning electron

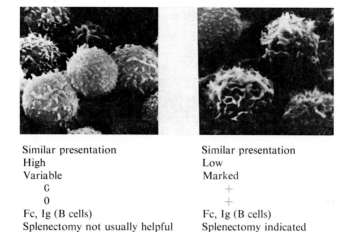

Clinical	Similar presentation	Similar presentation
WBC	High	Low
Splenomegaly	Variable	Marked
Phagocytosis	0	+
Acid phosphatase	0	+
Surface markers	Fc, Ig (B cells)	Fc, Ig (B cells)
Treatment	Splenectomy not usually helpful	Splenectomy indicated

FIG. 2. Clinical-pathological correlation: a comparison of the characteristics of chronic lymphatic leukaemia (left) and hairy-cell leukaemia (right).

microscope, it has been shown that certain patients with leukaemia have cells with different morphological characteristics and, further, that the structural differences can be correlated with functional variations and carry important prognostic and therapeutic implications (Fig. 2). The functional determination of structure is not a concept confined to the biological sciences. With the increasing sophistication of computers, it has now become a practical, indeed an economic necessity to verify how a system functions before the actual hardware is built. P. E. Haggerty put the matter provocatively when he said 'manual approaches to design with test by trial and error are no longer tenable. It takes, as it were, a computer to design a computer' (personal communication). Successive approximations are not enough.

In some instances, the time between recognition of the structural and functional components of a newly discovered biological system may be incredibly swift. In 1965 and 1966, intranuclear inclusions were observed in the glial cells of patients with subacute sclerosing leucoencephalitis.[32, 33]. Filamentous tubules 17–23 nanometres in diameter were observed, strongly suggesting that these cells had been infected with measles virus.[32, 33] In 1967 Connolly and his colleagues looked for and found antibodies and antigens to measles virus in patients with the disease.[34]

The final and perhaps the most important point I want to raise is that, although an approach to biological understanding from the vantage point of either structure or function may be rewarding, as biological phenomena are increasingly understood at the molecular level the differences between structure and function become vanishingly small.

Another striking structure–function relationship in the virus field is the recent demonstration by Scheid and Choppin[35] that proteolytic cleavage of one of the two glycoproteins that form the projections on the surfaces of para-influenza viruses, such as Sendai virus, activates the infectivity of the virus and its ability to cause cell fusion and haemolysis. Proteolytic cleavage is not required for the assembly of the virus particle, but only for the activation of these biological properties. This cleavage requires the presence of a host cell protease; thus the host range and tissue or organ tropism of these viruses is entirely dependent on the availability in the host tissue of a protease capable of activating the virus. Further, Scheid and Choppin[35] have isolated mutants which are activated by proteases other than those which activate the wild-type virus. This raises the possibility that when such mutants emerge under natural conditions the virus may infect an organ, such as the brain in leucoencephalitis or the pancreas in diabetes, which is not usually infected by the wild-type virus. Finally, the failure of an infective virus to form when there is no appropriate protease in the tissue may explain how these viruses can persist even when there is no virus production, a situation which is becoming increasingly implicated in the aetiology of chronic diseases.

Recently Choppin in New York[36] and Klenk in Giessen[37] have shown that the infectivity of influenza virus is activated by a conformational change in a glycoprotein, haemagglutinin, on the virus surface—a change resulting from a specific proteolytic cleavage of this protein by the host.

When, in addition to the above examples, one considers that a single base change in one codon may result in a single amino acid substitution in a protein which can so alter function that an easily recognizable clinical disease can be detected, the difference between structure and function is clearly more operational than real.

Structure and function should not stand apart; they should successively approximate, conjoin and unite to help us towards the common goal of understanding, at the most basic level, the pathogenesis of disease. For this forms the only sure basis for a rational study of disease; without it prevention and treatment is empirical, and the intellectual cohesion and unity of science is artificially distorted and depreciated.

The importance of understanding pathogenic mechanisms is beginning to overshadow the classic structure–function relationship. The immunologists are savaging the nephrologists. Viruses and infectious agents are everywhere— sometimes useful, sometimes harmful, forever interacting and even joining forces with the host they will soon embarrass. The delicate and harmonious and reassuring illusion of health is easily and unpredictably transformed into disease, and there is little we can do about it. The yardsticks of structure and function are crude and of limited usefulness when structure or function are fixed neither in time nor space. Structures fall apart, and refuse to function; functional disarray leads to structural perturbations. Structure and function are biologically inseparable. Though we may elect to study them individually, the fascination is to understand their interaction as we try to comprehend disease at the molecular level. Once we understand pathogenesis we can move on to one of the most important medical problems of today, namely prevention. For the molecular level of understanding in medicine is intrinsically no more interesting or more important than an understanding of the complexities of the whole organism interacting with an ever-changing environment.

I would like to end with an apologia. The permanently conjectural nature of scientific knowledge is inevitable but not discouraging. Even those things that I have said which I believe are true are probably half-truths, and the half-truths will probably be sunk without trace by my colleagues at this symposium. But let me end by paraphrasing a quotation from the pre-Socratic philosopher Xenophanes, a favourite of Karl Popper's, by saying: even if by chance I were to utter the truth, I would not know it; the final truth is after all but a woven web of guesses.[38]

ACKNOWLEDGEMENTS

This paper was the outcome of discussions with many colleagues at Cornell University Medical College and The Rockefeller University. I should particularly like to express my appreciation to H. G. Kunkel, Purnell Choppin, Peter Lachmann, Moran Campbell and John Dickinson with whom I discussed these ideas, and to Shu Man Fu, who discussed with me the work referred to in Fig. 2.

Discussion

Black: Dr Bearn's paper admirably complements Dr Eisenberg's paper in that it has shown us the strengths and the occasional weaknesses of the organic model, in particular its incompleteness.

Randle: The example of diabetes points up a number of problems. The discovery of insulin may have hindered diabetes research, perhaps because of its obvious efficacy in the juvenile form. People tended to say that diabetics already had the benefit of insulin and that research in diabetes is less urgent than research into some other diseases. The renewed interest in diabetes which has developed over the past twenty years is perhaps based partly on rising expectations of quality of life and partly on the growing awareness of diabetic complications and the failure of current methods of treatment of diabetes to prevent their appearance and development. It is also interesting to note that it took a war and the introduction of food rationing to provide hard information about the incidence of diabetes in the United Kingdom. This perhaps emphasizes that one can only gain limited information about the natural history of the disease from patients in hospital with diabetes.

Diabetes is *par excellence* a condition in which the distinction between disease and illness is important, as Dr Eisenberg has emphasized. Diabetes can exist as a chemical disease without any clear evidence of illness, and the benefits of treating mild chemical diabetes have still to be established.

It has been difficult to prove that diabetes is due to insulin deficiency and it is only within the present decade that there has been general acceptance of the view that insulin secretion is defective in nearly all diabetic patients. Thus there has been an interval of about forty-five years from the discovery of insulin to emergence of the view that defective secretion of the hormone is the rule in clinical diabetes. The emergence of this view has been important because it has focused attention on possible causes of β-cell damage or necrosis and on such processes as virus infection and autoimmunity. In other words classical lines of thought on the pathology of cell dysfunction and death are now being applied with enthusiasm to the pancreatic β-cell. The emergence of this view has also focused attention on the possibility that complications of diabetes may be due to inadequate insulin therapy. Insulin treatment of diabetes in its present form is a poor substitute for the minute-by-minute release of insulin by a healthy β-cell. One answer is the use of high technology for therapeutic research through the development of islet transplantation of the artificial pancreas. Although these developments may not be generally applicable as methods of treatment they may establish whether more physiological methods of insulin replacement can prevent complications.

Research into diabetes has perhaps not been helped by the creation of diabetic clinics. Clinics tend to be large and properly concentrated on the delivery of health care and they are perhaps not the milieu in which research can flourish. The formation of diabetic associations composed of diabetic patients, doctors, scientists and ancillary professions has however been helpful. Such associations can assist in the identification of special groups of patients who have a particular contribution to make to our understanding of the aetiology of diabetes. One can instance the value of identical twins, one of whom is diabetic and the other not, in studies of underlying genetic variations and their impact on the development of the disease.

Archibald Garrod recognized sixty or seventy years ago that diabetes is not an inborn error of metabolism. Diabetes appears to be one of those diseases in which susceptibility may be inherited but where environmental factors may lead to the onset of disease or illness. Perhaps genetic susceptibility should be added to disease and to illness to form a triad whose interrelations will have to be considered. The implications for health care would be considerable if there should be a case for advising restrictions for people with a particular genetic background.

Saracci: Dr Bearn's point about inferring causation from correlations recalls a problem familiar to the epidemiologist. Firstly, an intrinsic limitation of all classical clinico-pathological correlations lies in the very nature of the data, which are in fact observational, not experimental. In pathology, as in epidemiology or sociology, inferring causes from observations alone is a delicate and risky exercise. For example, at autopsy coronary thrombosis and myocardial infarction run together: does the thrombus cause the infarction, or does the infarct come first, with the circulation slowing down and thrombosis following, or are both caused by a third cause which affects blood-clotting properties on one side and myocardial vulnerability on the other? The mere fact of the observed association is compatible with all three causal sequences and external information is required to settle the question.

Secondly, inferring causation assumes that there is such a thing as a cause. I do not wish to slide into a philosophical argument, but surely what one defines as a cause is a function of the level of observation? At the macroscopic level, working in certain dye factories is a cause of bladder cancer; at the level of the portal of entry into the body, β-naphthylamine is a cause; at the cellular level, the hydroxylamine metabolite of β-naphthylamine is a cause. This has important consequences for the relationship between research and practice.

Once a causal association has been firmly established at one level of observation, research at more analytical levels (e.g. molecular) should continue but at the same time plans for preventive and corrective interventions must start immediately. The history of public health provides numerous examples of the benefits deriving from this approach.

Burgen: No system of medicine is tenable if it proposes no causality, Dr Saracci. But causality is a complicated matter and should not be treated as though there were simple one-to-one causal relations between things. We have to deal with hierarchies of causality all the time and in therapeutics of course everyone is familiar with this. Symptomatic treatment is really dealing with causality at a rather low level in the hierarchy, and one hopes, for instance, that chemotherapy of bacterial diseases deals with causality at a much higher level. In the whole consideration of pathogenesis and treatment one is always considering causal relationships, and where one cannot consider them there is utter chaos.

Dollery: We all seem to agree that man is a complex chemical engine. As Dr Bearn implied, the way this chemical engine is constituted largely determines its responses. But it is a programmable engine too, so its education, training and total experience determine its responses. Its responses are also determined by the environment, both in physical and social terms. Those were the four components of Dr Eisenberg's argument. I agree with Dr Eisenberg that tackling a particular illness or disease, which is what we as doctors are concerned with doing, must depend on us assessing which condition we can most usefully tackle at a particular time. Is it manipulation of the physical environment, or of the social environment, or of the totality of experience, that is the best thing to do at any particular time, or should one do something about the structure of the machine instead? As western societies develop a more uniform physical and social environment, it seems to me that the expression of disease and illness becomes more and more determined by the structure of the machine. In other words the relative importance of biochemical mechanisms has increased, not decreased. Our perception of the environmental and social factors may well have heightened in recent times but I think that their relative importance may be declining. Diseases like tuberculosis, or some of the grosser forms of environmental pollution, were much worse in the past than they are now, despite what the environmentalists would have us think. We can probably do more about the chemical structure of the machine than about its social environment or its programming.

We are of course considering this from the standpoint of medical practice, but nobody here would hold that medical practice is the only thing relevant to health and disease. Environment, political action and social factors are in many cases more important. In the past the general improvement in health has been due to these factors more than to what doctors have done. But now we have to consider what we can do about our part of the problem. In that sense I think Dr Bearn hit the nail very much on the head. The failures that happen now, such as hypertensive patients not taking their medicine, do not mean that the biological side has failed. Maybe someone will devise a chemical way of controlling hypertension that uses one pill or one injection on one occasion and then keeps the blood pressure down for good. That would get over that difficulty. We have not run out of ideas on the biochemical side.

Fliedner: You imply that we should look at human beings as 'systems', Dr Dollery. Perhaps the question should be, is there a disease of the system termed a human being, or are there conditions which we interpret as being harmful to the system, which we then term 'diseases'? Would it not be better to define the health problem that a person has? It is a health problem that we should try to characterize in physical terms, in psychological terms and perhaps in social terms. We cannot really distinguish which of the three is the most important.

We should also discuss the detrimental effect that Vesalius had on medicine, ending in Virchow's concept of cellular pathology. This has brought us the artificial separation of organs which may or may not have any meaning with respect to the malfunctioning of the system. I would be happy if we were to return to the concept of the human being as a whole and not as a composite of millions of cells or a couple of organs. From that point of view it becomes important to characterize also the role of medical research with respect to the qualitative as well as the quantitative aspects of the system called a human being.

References

[1] BRIGHT, R. (1827) *Reports of Medical Cases, Selected with a View to Illustrating the Symptoms and Cure of Diseases by a Reference to Morbid Anatomy*, Longman, London

[2] MORGAGNI, G. B. (1761) *De Sedibus, et Causis Morborum per Anatomen Indagatis Libri Quinique*, Venetiis, typog. Remondiniana

[3] BOISSIER DE SAUVAGES DE LA CROIX, F. (1768) *Nosologia Methodica, Sistens Morborum Classes, Genera et Species* (5 vols.), Amstelodami, Frat. de Tournes

[4] BICHÂT, M. F. X. (1800) *Recherches Physiologiques sur la Vie et la Mort*, Brosson, Garbon et Cie, Paris

[5] VON MERING, J. & MINKOWSKI, O. (1890) Diabetes mellitus nach Pankreasextirpation. *Archiv für Experimentelle Pathologie und Pharmakologie 26*, 371-87 (quoted from Major, R. H. (1965) *Classic Descriptions of Disease*, 3rd edn., Thomas, Springfield, Ill.)

[6] OPIE, E. L. (1907) On the relation of chronic interstitial pancreatitis to the islands of Langerhans and to diabetes mellitus. *Journal of Experimental Medicine 5*, 397-428

[7] SHARPEY-SCHAFER, Sir E. A. (1916) *The Endocrine Organs, An Introduction to the Study of Internal Secretion*, Longmans, Green, London

[8] BANTING, F. G. & BEST, C. H. (1922) The internal secretion of the pancreas. *Journal of Laboratory and Clinical Medicine 7*, 251-66

[9] DE DUVE, C. (1952) Glucagon, the hyperglycemic-glycogenolytic factor of the pancreas. *Acta Physiologica et Pharmacologia Neerlandica, 2*, 311-314

[10] CUATRECASAS, P. (1975) Hormone – receptor interactions and the plasma membrane, in *Cell Membranes, Biochemistry, Cell Biology & Pathology*, pp. 177-184, H.P. Publishing Co., New York

[11] FLIER, J. S., KAHN, C. R., ROTH, J. & BAR, R. S. (1975) Antibodies that impair insulin receptor binding in an unusual diabetic syndrome with severe insulin resistance. *Science (Washington, D.C.) 190*, 63-65

[12] MCKUSICK, V. A. (1975) *Mendelian Inheritance in Man: Autosomal Dominant, Autosomal Recessive & X-linked Phenotypes*, Johns Hopkins Press, Baltimore

[13] HARRIS, H. (1966) Enzyme polymorphism in man. *Proceedings of the Royal Society of London B Biological Sciences 164*, 298-310

[14] HARRIS, H. (1971) Annotation: polymorphism & protein evolution. The neutral mutation-random drift hypothesis. *Journal of Medical Genetics 8*, 444-452

[15] Editorial (1975) Heritability of diabetes. *British Medical Journal, 4*, 127-128

[16] MAUGH, T. H. (1975) Diabetes: epidemiology suggests a viral connection. *Science (Washington, D.C.) 188*, 347-351

[17] KOENIG, R. J. & CERAMI, A. (1975) Synthesis of hemoglobin A_{Ic} in normal and diabetic mice: potential model of basement membrane thickening. *Proceedings of the National Academy of Sciences of the United States of America 72*, 3687-3691

[18] LEJEUNE, J. (1975) Sur les mécanismes de la spéciation. *Comptes Rendus des Séances de la Société de Biologie et ses Filiales, 169*, 828-844

[19] PENROSE, L. S. & SMITH, G. F. (1966) *Down's Anomaly*. Churchill, London

[20] WOODFORD, F. P. & BEARN, A. G. (1970) A critical examination of some reported biochemical abnormalities in mongolism. *Annals of the New York Academy of Sciences 171*, 551-558

[21] HARRIS, H. (1975) *The Principles of Human Biochemical Genetics*, 2nd edn., North-Holland, Amsterdam

[22] BERGSMA, D. (ed.) (1975) *New Chromosomal and Malformation Syndromes (Birth Defects Original Article Ser. No. 11-5)*, Stratton Intercontinental, New York

[23] JEROME, H., LEJEUNE, J. & TURPIN, R. (1960) Etude de l'excrétion urinaire de certaines métabolites du tryptophane chez les enfants mongoliens. *Comptes Rendus Hebdomadaires des Séances de l'Académie des Sciences 251*, 474-476

[24] FORD, E. B. (1940) The new systematics, in *Polymorphism and Taxonomy* (Huxley, J., ed.), pp. 493-513, Clarendon Press, Oxford

[25] ALLISON, A. C. (1954) Protection afforded by sickle cell trait against subtertian malarial infection. *British Medical Journal 1*, 290-294

[26] MILLER, L. H., MASON, S. J., DVORAK, J. A., McGINNIS, M. H. & ROTHMAN, I. K. (1975) Erythrocyte receptors for (*Plasmodium knowlesi*) malaria: Duffy blood group determinants. *Science (Washington, D.C.) 189*, 561-563

[27] PARKER, W. C. & BEARN, A. G. (1962) Additional genetic variation of human serum transferrin. *Science (Washington, D.C.) 137*, 854-855

[28] HARVEY, W. (1628) *Exercitatio de Motu Cordis et Sanguinis in Animalibus*, Francofurti, sumpt. Guilielmi Fitzeri

[29] MALPIGHI, M. (1661) *De Pulmonibus Observationes Anatomicae*, Bononiae

[30] EHRLICH, P. (1900) On immunity with special reference to cell life. *Proceedings of the Royal Society (London) 66*, 424 (from Talmage, D. W. & Cohen, E. P. (1965) in *Immunological Diseases* (Samter, M., ed.), p. 89, Little, Brown, Boston)

[31] KUNKEL, H. G. (1975) Surface markers of human lymphocytes. *Johns Hopkins Medical Journal 137*, 216-223

[32] BOUTEILLE, M., FONTAINE, C., VEDRENNE, C. & DELARUE, J. (1965) Sur un cas d'encéphalite subaiguë à inclusions. Etude anatomoclinique et ultrastructurale. *Revue Neurologique (Paris) 113*, 454-458

[33] TELLEZ-NAGEL, I. & HARTER, D. H. (1966) Subacute sclerosing leukoencephalitis: ultrastructure of intranuclear and intracytoplasmic inclusions. *Science (Washington. D.C.) 154*, 899-901

[34] CONNOLLY, J. H., ALLEN, L. V., HURWITZ, L. J. & MILLAR, J. H. O. (1967) Measles-virus antibody and antigen in subacute sclerosing panencephalitis. *Lancet 1*, 542-544

[35] SCHEID, A. & CHOPPIN, P. W. (1975) Activation of cell fusion & infectivity by proteolytic cleavage of a Sendai virus glycoprotein, in *Proteases and Biological Control* (Reich, E., Rifkin, D. B. & Shaw, E., eds.), pp. 645-659, Cold Spring Harbor Laboratory, New York

[36] LAZAROWITZ, S. G. & CHOPPIN, P. W. (1976) Enhancement of the infectivity of influenza A and B viruses by proteolytic cleavage of the hemagglutinin polypeptide. *Virology 68*, 440-454

[37] KLENK, H. D., ROTT, R., ORLICH, M. & BLÖDORN, J. (1976) Activation of influenza A viruses by trypsin treatment. *Virology 68*, 426-439

[38] XENOPHANES [quoted from Popper, K. (1971) in *Modern British Philosophy* (Magee, B., ed.), p. 78, St Martin's Press, New York]

Clinical science

E. J. M. CAMPBELL

Department of Medicine, McMaster University, Hamilton, Ontario

Abstract The most obvious achievements of clinical science have been in the elucidation of symptoms and signs and the patterns of disordered function due to failure of the organs or to nutritional disturbances. The benefits of clinical research are both direct—through improved practice—and indirect—through improved teaching and contributions to biological science.

It is suggested that the clinical scientist, experienced in both clinical and research work, has a potential not to be expected from collaboration between non-scientific clinicians and non-clinical scientists.

Problems which particularly affect clinical research include: ethics; difficulty in being experimentally rigorous; the need to be opportunistic; dependence on transient workers; excessive concern with the end stages of irreversible disease; triviality; uncritical and premature imitation of research in practice.

Clinical science is always threatened by a tendency for its problems to be regarded simply as applied problems of basic science.

The roles of the clinical scientist should include: elucidating clinical phenomena, about most of which we remain very ignorant; collaboration with basic scientists on the one hand and with community scientists on the other; and clarifying the description and analysis of illnesses.

I have taken as my subject the study of the functional (physiological, bio-chemical, etc.) disorders observed in sick people. Clinical science often also requires the study of structural, genetic and other matters and its pursuit may well require studies of normal people and of animals, but I think the focus I have adopted will be sensibly separate from those of my neighbouring speakers.

Although there have always been clinical scientists, as a breed they became established only within this century with the founding by Sir Thomas Lewis and others of the Medical Research Society and, in the United States, with the foundation of the American Society for Clinical Investigation.[1]

The best case for clinical science being of benefit to practice would probably

LIST 1

Symptoms and signs

General:	Fever, weight loss or gain, thirst, pain
Cardiorespiratory symptoms:	Angina pectoris and pleuritic pain, dyspnoea, cyanosis, haemorrhage, oedema, palpitation, high and low blood pressure
Alimentary symptoms:	Hunger, dysphagia, vomiting, diarrhoea and constipation
Urinary symptoms:	Frequency, polyuria, dysuria, proteinuria
Neurology:	Either all or none—by that I mean that nearly all the physiology or functional anatomy underlying the practice of neurology has been learned by clinical scientists. However, today much of it bears little relationship to the physiology of the physiologists

LIST 2

The functional syndromes

Body fluids:	Water depletion and overload; Electrolyte (notably Na^+ and K^+) depletion and overload; Acidosis and alkalosis
Blood:	Anaemias; Haemostatic and thrombotic disorders
Heart and circulation:	Shock; High and low blood pressure; Congestive heart failure; Rhythm disorders
Respiration:	Anoxia and cyanosis; Airways obstruction; Respiratory failure
Kidney:	Renal failure; Nephrotic syndrome; Tubular disorders
Gut:	Maldigestion and malabsorption
Liver:	Jaundice; Liver cell failure; Portal hypertension; Porto-systemic shunting
Connective tissue:	Osteoporosis and osteomalacia
Endocrinology:	Over-activity, under-activity or abnormal activity of all the endocrine glands (including the gonads)
Metabolism:	Diabetes mellitus
Neurology:	See List 1.

be made in two directions: first, in elucidating the way disease processes cause symptoms and signs (List 1); and secondly, in describing and elucidating patterns of disordered function which, although they may have multiple causes, nevertheless require recognition and management in their own right (such patterns are sometimes called the functional syndromes) (List 2). I shall not go through the lists in detail for a number of reasons. First, their chief value is as indications of the sort of topics I am talking about. Secondly, I think the benefit of most of the examples is both unprovable and self-evident. Finally, even if those benefits were provable, it might be argued that the useful days of clinical science are over and one should be more interested in the future. I would rather spend my time on this future than on a historic defence.

Therefore, having put the lists before you, I propose to tackle the following major topics:
(1) The necessary conditions for the advance implied in the items;
(2) The ways in which such research has been of benefit;
(3) Problems, limitations and criticisms;
(4) Present status and future roles.

THE NECESSARY CONDITIONS FOR THE DISCOVERIES IMPLIED IN THE TWO LISTS

The discoveries implied in Lists 1 and 2 all required minds interested in the way the body functions to apply themselves to a clinical problem. Sometimes this application was achieved by collaboration of 'scientist' and 'clinician', but usually it was achieved because one man was both.

Although research on obvious problems may go well by collaboration, as a Popperian I believe that the peculiar alchemy leading to a conjecture (an intuition, an idea) needs the intimacy of one mind. To drive the point further I will risk a boast: I believe that my good fortune in having the requisite grasp of physiology and sufficient clinical experience enabled me to have ideas that would not have come from collaboration between a better physiologist and a better clinician. I am not claiming any merit for the ideas—I am just trying to account for them!

Trotter makes the point against dependency on collaboration between scientists and clinicians on a grander scale:

'In 1754 Dr. James Lind, in his *Treatise on the Scurvy*, showed what scurvy is due to, and advised its treatment, as we do to-day, by lemon juice. To give some sort of a time scale for the effects of this disclosure I may mention a small scrap of naval history. The Lords of the Admiralty, concerned at the existence of an agency for the destruction of seamen more effective than the enemy's guns, and with the deference for hygiene characteristic of all military bodies, adopted Lind's recommendations for the Navy after an interval of only forty years. But it was 150 years before physiology, having taken that time to come round to it, discovered the existence of vitamin C. Thus it took not forty years but a century and a half for one of the clearest and most direct hints for medicine to produce an effect in the physiological world.

'Such phenomena in the natural history of knowledge are of course in no way a reproach to physiology. It was in the structure of events that an experience of medicine, which now seems so rich with intimations, should fail for so long to reach and inspire the physiologist; it was also no less in the structure of events that those engaged in medicine and fully open to these hints should have neither the training nor the inclination that could have led them to submit the familiar facts to experimental analysis'.[2]

By contrast one may refer to the comparative speed of the insulin story. Platt[3] included it in his list of discoveries not made by clinical scientists but, as Good[4] pointed out, although the facilities used by Banting and Best were in physiology, the problem and the drive to solve it came from clinical science.

THE WAY THESE ADVANCES HAVE BEEN OF BENEFIT TO MEDICINE

Directly, by improvement in clinical technique

Symptoms, signs and investigations are more useful if they are understood. At its nicest, this sort of research may be almost 'self-destructive'. Thus, the understanding, while it may have come through invasive techniques, lessens the need for these techniques. *Examples:* the contribution of cardiac catheterization to clinical examinations of the heart; the way the protean manifestations of liver failure or the various endocrine disturbances have been made coherent; the way renal biopsy has improved our ability to interpret proteinuria.

The conditions in the second list are entities whose management is improved by recognition of their common features whatever the cause.

Indirectly, by their contributions to biology

Some whole disciplines such as physiology and biochemistry which are now independent were begun by clinicians. That is history. There are however some sciences which continue to depend on an intimate relationship with clinical research. *Examples:* human physiology, clinical pharmacology, immunology, haematology, endocrinology, genetics.

Through education

Most of us think it desirable that doctors should know how the body works. I further believe that clinical scientists can teach how the body works in both health and disease in a way which is at least complementary and often superior to the usual arrangement of the curriculum in which the academic physiologists are followed by clinicians concerned almost exclusively with practice.

Certain features or principles, although part of the canon of classical physiology originating with such people as Bernard, Sherrington, Haldane and Barcroft are now most characteristic of the stories (models, paradigms) of clinical scientists. Let me mention three: integration, pattern, capacity. The need to have an *integrative* view of the organism as well as understanding of its mechanisms is naturally always asserting itself in clinical science. The *patterns* of disordered function, such as the several syndromes of respiratory failure, of liver failure or of renal failure, are illustrative of the differing problems posed by various environmental and metabolic needs. *Examples:* the syndromes of respiratory failure depend on the physicochemical differences between oxygen and carbon dioxide; the syndromes of liver failure depend on the different demands posed by the metabolism of different carbohydrates, fats and proteins; the syndromes of renal failure depend on the chemical and environmental differences between water and various electrolytes.

Finally, most of our understanding of the functional *capacity* of the various organs and systems comes from clinical science, because the effects of disease on such capacities are particularly compelling problems for clinicians. Furthermore, the procedures required to stress and measure the effects on the organs of man are more acceptable to clinicians.

PROBLEMS, DIFFICULTIES AND CRITICISMS

In this section I shall begin with problems which are inherent in clinical science and move on to those which are accidental unfortunate consequences.

Ethics. Much attention has been devoted to the spectre of the clinical scientist treating his patients as guinea pigs. I shall make only two points. First, while applauding the Helsinki and similar declarations, I think they can only remind—they cannot relieve—the clinical scientist of the conflict between scientific curiosity and professional responsibility. This is in a way a reinforcement of my earlier assertion that it is better for one man to be both the clinician and the scientist. Fortunately, the resolution can often be achieved by reasoning and ingenuity. I think this is one way in which the good clinical scientist —the physician–scholar— can be distinguished. Secondly, I am much more worried about the harm done by the premature use of investigations and treatments which should really still be regarded as in the research stage by investigators or clinicians whose critical standards are lower than they ought to be.

Rigorous experimental design is difficult and may be unattainable because for clinical or ethical reasons one cannot control or measure all the variables.

Opportunism. Although many of the problems tackled by clinical scientists occur in patients with common or chronic and stable conditions, often they come up unexpectedly because, of course, illness is unpredictable. These circumstances make research planning, experimental design and even ethics difficult.

Dependence on transient workers. Although continuity of direction may come from established senior people, most of the actual work is usually done by transient workers,[5] who must hope for results from their labour in a year or two. This expectation puts a premium on industry rather than originality and limits the length and depth of research projects.

Let me expand on these problems by mentioning difficulties at both ends of the time scale of illness. First, elucidation of acute problems such as acute cardiorespiratory emergencies is hard work. The front-line staff are junior, the senior people cannot easily hold themselves in readiness for the unexpected, the clinical and ethical situation is nerve-racking. Secondly, the study of illness which unfolds over the years requires a build-up and continuity of practice which make extraordinary demands, similar to doing experiments which last many years.

Much clinical research is concerned with the end-stages of disease. The reserves of the organs and systems of the body are so great that their dysfunction only becomes manifest when disease is advanced. It is therefore not surprising that clinical research of this sort has not offered much to mild, preventable or curable disease. But I would make two points in partial rebuttal of this criticism. First, the manifestations of illness are not peculiar to rare or irreversible illnesses; lessons learned from the rare usually elucidate the commonplace. Secondly, modern techniques allow us increasingly to study the less ill—and in their usual environments, not just in hospital.

Clinical research too readily becomes trivial. The proliferation of new things to measure or new ways of measuring old things encourages much purposeless work and nourishes a flourishing secondary industry of comparison between measurements.

The frontier between research and practice is vague and there is a danger of premature and uncritical imitation of research in practice which can be expensive, confusing and even risky. This unfortunate consequence is partly the fault of the research worker who naturally wants to sell his product, and partly the fault of the clinician whose sales resistance is too low.

Perhaps I could link the last four or five problems by cynically wondering how often and how quickly this year's ethically questionable experiment becomes a routine—even obligatory—procedure.

There are dangers in 'lumping'. Although I have claimed that the patterns of disordered function in List 2 require management in their own right, there is a danger that 'giving the thing a name' can inhibit research and also cause what must be essentially symptomatic treatment to substitute entirely for more rational measures. *Examples:* acidosis and alkalosis; arterial hypoxaemia, acute hypotension (e.g. after myocardial infarction). I regret to admit that I think the treatments for such as these are often technically meddlesome, biologically myopic and clinically superficial.

PAST, PRESENT AND FUTURE

To a romantic it may seem that there was a golden age in clinical science (which ended just before one began one's own work) during which there was a happy coincidence of favourable circumstances. There were plenty of soluble problems. Physiological (biochemical, pharmacological, etc.) knowledge and techniques had reached a point at which they were applicable to clinical problems but the techniques were still inexpensive and simple so that a clinician with at the most an ingenious technician could learn a lot—i.e. there was little technical trouble. These problems were of direct importance to the individual patient—i.e. there was little ethical trouble. The clinical and scientific training of a clinical investigator could be blended in a mixed experience lasting two or three years after he completed his junior house appointments and was good for him whatever his subsequent career, even if it were to be purely clinical, i.e. there was little manpower trouble.

Our seniors might accept that romantic view provided it was tempered by recognition that problems which seem obvious and soluble afterwards are not so at the time, and by appreciation of the difficulties they faced, which are much less today, over such matters as jobs, remuneration, resources and lack of respect (both by clinicians and 'basic' scientists).

It might be thought that today the frontiers of research have moved on. To make progress requires prolonged training in some basic science, membership of a research team and expensive facilities. I think this view reflects a 'snob rating' which ranks sciences according to their level of 'basicity'. Thus biochemistry rates higher than physiology, biophysics and molecular biology rate higher than biochemistry, and so on. Acceptance of this view implies that the only respectable direction of science is 'reductionist'—that is, explaining phenomena in terms of more basic knowledge. The medical curriculum, the reward structure of the scientific community, the contents of journals of clinical research, all bear witness to: 'the more basic, the better'. I think this attitude must be challenged. Although strengthened by roots in more basic sciences, the health of a science really depends on the rigour of its own empiricism.

The need to resist the tendency to reduce clinical problems to problems of applied science and the need to assert the legitimacy of clinical science is not new. This need has been cogently argued over the years by many of the greatest clinical scientists (Meltzer[6]; Cohn[7]; Pickering[8]; Seldin[9]). But the basic sciences are so much easier on the nerves, and more glamorous, that I fancy the need for clinical science to be assertive will be endless.

THE FUTURE ROLES OF CLINICAL RESEARCH

I see three roles of clinical research which are non-controversial and un-changing and I am going to add one which is not given the recognition I think it deserves.

(1) To do its proper thing

There is an abundance of clinical problems calling for research—but they must be seen as clinical problems which, though they may require the application of 'basic' science, are not just applied problems in the relevant science. *Examples:* we remain very ignorant about some of the commonest symptoms, such as pain, fatigue, anorexia, obesity, weight loss, dyspnoea, cough and sputum, constipation and diarrhoea. (The fact that most of these examples also occur in my first list should occasion no surprise.)

Our ignorance is often most apparent and irritating with regard to the mechanisms of these symptoms but, to reinforce the point I was making above, there are other levels calling for research which I suspect will become more pressing rather than less should we elucidate the mechanisms. *Examples:* were the neuroanatomy and neurophysiology of pain or dyspnoea to be worked out, I am sure we would then perceive more precisely numerous problems arising from the variability in these symptoms between conditions, between people, between responses to different treatments. And I will go further: I do not believe that pain or dyspnoea—not to mention lassitude or debility—will be 'explicable' in purely neurophysiological terms.

(2) To collaborate with the basic sciences

Putting partisanship aside, the 'relevance' of the basic sciences and the health of clinical science require that the two keep closely in touch. The clinical scientist also has an essential role as interpreter and honest broker between the basic scientist and the clinician.

(3) To collaborate with epidemiologists and clinical trialists

It is fashionable to compare the contributions of clinical science unfavourably with those of epidemiology, and particularly with the controlled clinical trial (e. g. Platt[3]). If such comparisons are made in a spirit of camaraderie like that between medicine and surgery or between units in the armed services, they can be good fun but, also like these examples, if carried too far they can cause unnecessary friction and weakness in the face of a common enemy.

Although epidemiology and so on are very powerful disciplines, they need the collaboration of clinical scientists. Without it their studies may produce crude or irrelevant results.[10] *Examples:* (1) (A personal one): about fifteen years ago, I was asked to participate in a multi-centre controlled trial of the value of tracheostomy in respiratory failure in chest disease. Most of the hospitals could not measure blood gases so these were to be ignored. In retrospect I think I was correct in refusing to take part in this massive assault and was better employed in going on sniping in my own way. (2) (Also personal but not so directly): I am at present on the fringe of the flurry of interest in exercise and heart disease. 'Will exercise prevent recurrence of myocardial infarction?' Studies meant to answer such a question are liable to be gross. Firstly, the effects of myocardial infarction on the way the heart responds to exercise may be very variable. Patients with one sequela may be cured by exercise, with another they may be killed. Secondly, there are other things besides the heart which are usually in poor shape in middle-aged western men who have had heart attacks. Thirdly, we have little information on the 'dose-response characteristics' of exercise. Fourthly, exercise may well have beneficial effects which will not be revealed if recurrence is the sole criterion. Yet most of these studies include only a crude exercise test. (3) I suspect many clinicians share my concern that the studies (and the rhetoric) on the value of anti-coagulants in myocardial infarction ended in inconclusive boredom. While accepting the overall negative result we still suspect that better and more discriminating antithrombosis measures may be of value. History may have been unkind in its timing—as it would have been to a trial of liver in 'anaemia' before Addison or Minot and Murphy. (4) The early but well performed trials of corticosteroids and of cromoglycate in asthma nearly failed to detect the value of these substances.

(4) The need to improve the ways we describe and classify illness (nosology and taxonomy)

I am now going to tackle a fundamental problem which I think bedevils medicine in a way transcending my immediate terms of reference but which I think will be solved only by clinical scientists and will, in its solution, emphasize and increase their responsibility. It concerns the limited utility of the concept of 'A Disease'.

Dr Bearn[11] has already referred to the different bases—syndromal, structural, functional, genetic, etc.—by which Diseases may be characterized. It may be useful and I hope it is legitimate to regard the concept of 'A Disease' as a paradigm in the sense that Kuhn[12] uses the term. At its simplest, as reflected in our teaching and the composition of most textbooks, the paradigm of A Disease seems to me as follows:

A Disease is first recognized syndromally—a constellation of clinical features. The Disease has a cause (infective, nutritional, genetic, immunological, etc.); this cause produces characteristic structural changes which in turn cause characteristic functional disturbances which in turn produce the clinical manifestations. The elucidation of the causative, structural and functional changes may not come in any particular historical order but the paradigm has two characteristics: first, it is expected or at least hoped that the relations will be specific (unique cause, unique structural and functional changes belonging to one syndrome); secondly, as knowledge progresses, the defining characteristic is 'pushed to the left' in the sequence given above. In other words, a Disease will not be characterized in syndromal terms if it can be explained or defined in functional terms; a functional syndrome (e.g. diabetes, asthma) will not be left in these terms if it can be characterized structurally; and 'cause' takes priority over all. As witness, I could cite the avoidance of the term Disease, when, from the beginning, such specificity is unlikely (e.g. malabsorption syndrome, respiratory distress syndrome), or if it turns out not to be true (e.g. the demotion of angina pectoris from a disease to a syndrome).

Disease as a paradigm has at least two major unfortunate consequences. First, as Bearn pointed out (this volume, pp. 25–35),[11] the discovery of 'cause' may inhibit legitimate research at the other levels. Secondly, and I think much more persuasive and profound for both research and practice, the employment of the paradigm leads to confusing and even illegitimate discourse.

Let me try to clarify by giving some near-specific examples. It is no good reporting that a certain feature (clinical finding, test, chemical variable) is present in an observed proportion of the patients with A Disease unless a defining characteristic—not just a description of the condition—has been adopted. Many such studies are concerned with attempts to recognize the marginal case and it is, of course, in just such cases that attempts to use descriptions of the typical as definitions of the category break down. Such 'research' often drifts through triviality into tautology. After a few removes, the derivation of one feature is reported to be present in a high proportion of cases—the cases having been defined by the original feature.

Secondly, it is no good in research or practice asking 'either/or' questions unless the defining characteristic is in the same category of phenomena. *Examples:* distinguishing rheumatoid arthritis from systemic lupus erythematosus, asthma from chronic bronchitis, ulcerative colitis from Crohn's disease. (I am not questioning the practical—prognostic or therapeutic—end of such questions, particularly when they are asked about individual patients. I am only questioning the utility of The Disease as a means to the end.) As new levels of understanding increase or become more powerful (e.g. molecular biology, cellular physiology, genetics, immunology) the possibilities of confusion and non-communication will only increase if we try to conduct our discourses using the paradigm of The Disease. *Example:* recently I heard a world authority list eleven varieties or variations of what I shall call chronic semantic hepatitis. It was difficult to know whether any or all of them were legitimate variants or confusing synonyms. It did seem, however, that the terms were obscuring good attempts to progress along related but separate paths (aetiological, genetic, structural, biochemical, immunological, prognostic).

Most people deny that they use the term Disease in this way. They assert that it is merely a shorthand description and some people have explicitly (Scadding[13]) or implicitly (Feinstein[14]) attempted to adopt a purely nominalist stance on the use of Disease, but I have been doing some research on verbal habits which makes me sceptical about such assertions. The natural desire of a person, whether he be a patient or a doctor, to have explanations for illness has so encrusted Diseases with essentialist undertones that it will be difficult to re-order them to a nominalist role. However, the alternative—a new, separate terminology—is probably impracticable. I suspect that such developments as numerical taxonomy and the use of computers in decision-taking will force a quiet revolution and lead to Diseases being accepted as merely names.

If and when the revolution comes about, it will inevitably promote clinical science, because who other than the clinical scientists will be able to draw order out of the several categories of phenomena that make up the sick patient?

I will close with a passage from Trotter which elegantly summarizes what I have tried to say:

'Experiment in man, or direct experiment, limited in possibilities of application as it necessarily must be, is the one wholly unexceptionable method available for the solution of problems of human health and disease. Though its history is still very short, it has already proved remarkably fruitful. There can be no doubt that one of the chief duties before medicine at present is the exploitation of the method of direct experiment. The natural history of sciences, however, seems to indicate that a diet of pure experimentation in a limited field is not enough for permanent scientific health. If experimental medicine is to progress healthily it must have a full supply of ideas, and must know how to deal with them. Such a purpose can best be served by a close contact with the realities of clinical medicine'. (ref. 2, p. 126).

ACKNOWLEDGEMENT

I prepared this paper while holding a Josiah Macy Jr. Faculty Scholarship 1975-76 at The Royal Postgraduate Medical School, London.

References

1   AUSTIN, J. H. (1949) A brief sketch of the history of the American Society for Clinical Investigation. *Journal of Clinical Investigation 28*, 401-408
2   TROTTER, W. (1941) *The Collected Papers of Wilfred Trotter*, Oxford University Press, London
3   PLATT, LORD (1967) Medical science: master or servant? *British Medical Journal 4*, 439-444
4   GOOD, R. A. (1968) Keystones. *Journal of Clinical Investigation 47*, 1466-1471
5   PEART, W. S. (1958) Medical research and emigration. *Lancet 2*, 1232-1233
6   MELTZER, S. J. (1909) The science of clinical medicine: what it ought to be and the men to uphold it. *Journal of the American Medical Association 53*, 508-512
7   COHN, A. E. (1924) Purposes in medical research. *Journal of Clinical Investigation 1*, 1-11
8   PICKERING, G. W. (1949) The place of the experimental method in medicine. *Proceedings of the Royal Society of Medicine 42*, 229-234
9   SELDIN, D. W. (1966) Some reflections on the role of basic research and service in clinical departments. *Journal of Clinical Investigation 45*, 976-979
10 FLETCHER, C. M. (1963) Epidemiologist and clinical investigator. *Proceedings of the Royal Society of Medicine 56*, 851-858
11 BEARN, A. G. (1976) Structural determinants of disease and their contribution to clinical and scientific progress, in this volume, pp. 25-35
12 KUHN, T. S. (1970) *The Structure of Scientific Revolutions*, 2nd edn., University of Chicago Press, Chicago
13 SCADDING, J. G. (1967) Diagnosis: the clinician and the computer. *Lancet 2*, 877-882
14 FEINSTEIN, A. R. (1967) *Clinical Judgement*, Williams & Wilkins, Baltimore

This paper and the following one, by C. J. Dickinson, are discussed together on pp. 63–71

TABLE 1

Total number of papers in the four journals examined, and the percentage submitted from clinical and preclinical medical school departments, in 1956

	Total no. of papers examined	% from clinical depts	% from preclinical depts
Am. J. Physiol	444	8.6	60
J. Physiol. (Lond.)	231	8.9	66
J. Clin. Invest.	159	82	11
Clin. Sci.	61	85	10

that much of the best-planned clinical investigation done around 1955 will have been published in the *Journal of Clinical Investigation* in the USA and in *Clinical Science* in the UK. (In 1956 the title of the latter journal was not contaminated by the present curiously apologetic addition of 'Molecular Medicine'.) During 1956, 444 papers were published in the *American Journal of Physiology*[2] and 231 in the *Journal of Physiology*[3]; only about one-third as many papers were published in clinical research journals in that year (159 in the *Journal of Clinical Investigation*[4] and 61 in *Clinical Science*[5]). Table 1 shows, as percentages, the proportion of papers in each journal originating from clinical departments (e.g. medicine, surgery, pathology and allied departments of teaching and non-teaching hospitals), and the proportion coming from preclinical departments (e.g. physiology, biochemistry, pharmacology, anatomy). Work coming jointly from a preclinical and clinical department was scored as half in each category. The American and the British journals are closely similar and the only notable difference (the rather smaller proportion of papers in the *American Journal of Physiology*, compared with the *Journal of Physiology*, that come from preclinical departments of medical schools) is simply a reflection of the larger number of dedicated research institutes, such as the National Institutes of Health in the United States. Table 2 shows the average figures for

TABLE 2

Average numbers of papers coming from clinical and preclinical departments, published in 'physiological' and 'clinical' journals

	% from clinical depts	% from preclinical depts
'Physiological'	9	63
'Clinical'	83	11

TABLE 3

Analysis of papers in British and American journals coming from teaching and non-teaching hospitals

	Clinical departments	
	% from undergraduate teaching hospitals	% from non-teaching hospitals
American	91	9
British	88	12
All journals	90	10

all 'physiological' journals and for all 'clinical' journals in the two countries. There are very few preclinical departments outside medical schools and, in 1956 at least, all the published work in physiological journals which did *not* come from preclinical departments and research institutes came from the clinical departments of undergraduate teaching hospitals. The non-teaching hospitals supplied only a small proportion of the whole material published in 1956 (Table 3), and in proportion to the total numbers of medical staff the proportion must have been very small indeed.

As expected, most experiments and observations reported in journals of physiology were performed on animals, and most of those reported in clinical science journals were made on normal human subjects or on patients (Table 4). The apparent dearth of experimental work performed on man in physiological departments in the USA reflects, I imagine, the existence of the *Journal of Applied Physiology*, to which the UK has no exact counterpart. However, many of the papers published then and now in the *Journal of Applied Physiology* are in any case from clinical rather than preclinical departments. In 1956 there was still evidently a tradition of publishing quite a lot of work on the physiology of man in the *Journal of Physiology*. My brief scan through the titles of current

TABLE 4

Analysis of papers in the four journals, in 1956, derived from observations in man and in animals

	Animals %	Man %
Am. J. Physiol	99	1
J. Physiol. (Lond.)	81	19
J. Clin. Invest.	20	80
Clin. Sci.	9	91

articles in 1975 suggests that this relatively large proportion (19%) has now fallen about as low as it was in the *American Journal of Physiology*. Of the 19%, at least half came from clinical departments and were published in the *Journal of Physiology* presumably because their authors thought the work described was more appropriately published there. The scientific criteria for acceptance of papers in the two journals are not enormously different. The other point which emerges from Table 4 is that the *Journal of Clinical Investigation* accepted about one-fifth of papers based on animal work, which was in most cases manifestly relevant to clinical practice.

So far my analysis has been factual. The analysis which follows is necessarily subjective, but I hope you will accept my assurance that I have no particular axe to grind, and have published papers in both physiological and clinical journals.

The largest broad category of investigation reported (64% in clinical journals and 57% in physiological journals) might be described as the repetition of previously reported measurements, sometimes by improved techniques, often to resolve disputed or conflicting results from different laboratories. Another familiar type of investigation in this category is that in which an established but fairly new technique is applied to a new problem. An example from 1956 might be the use of electromyography of the calf and thigh muscles to investigate the effects of wearing high heels; another is the measurement of calf blood flow after surgical repair of the femoral artery. The first paper is in the *Journal of Physiology:* the second in *Clinical Science*. The second largest category (6% of clinical journal articles and 24% of physiological journal articles) was made up of descriptions of some previously unknown function or structure, often of a rather obscure or recondite nature. Only a small proportion of such papers came from clinical departments. In both types of journal there were a few papers describing new methodology and many describing new measurements. Sometimes a new technique is described at the same time as the striking results which its application brings. An example might be the first description of the hitherto unsuspected existence of cerebral autoregulation (in the cat) using a thermistor probe technique (in the *Journal of Physiology*). About 7% of papers in both the clinical and physiological journals were concerned with the effects of drugs, either of new drugs with physiologically interesting actions or of the more exotic effects or metabolism of old drugs. I imagine that this relative dearth of pharmacology reflects the existence of fundamental journals in that specialty on both sides of the Atlantic, and of general medical journals in which many clinical trials are reported. There was a surprisingly small category of papers stating hypotheses and then describing the experimental tests of the hypotheses. This exemplifies the truth of Medawar's contention that the scientific paper as usually presented is a fraud.[6] Authors tend to describe their research in a conventional way which makes the investigation sound dull and lifeless, even though the authors were in a high state of excitement at the time, thinking of all sorts of hypotheses and putting them to all sorts of tests.

The final and most subjective stage of the analysis was to assess how much of the research done around 1954/55 and reported in 1956 has had and continues to have an influence on medical practice today. I must confess to an initial prejudice that possibly very little work done twenty years ago could still be said to be clinically relevant, but I was quite astounded by the scope and continuing clinical relevance of much that was published twenty years ago. Table 5 gives a list of some clinically relevant papers published in physiological

TABLE 5

Clinically relevant articles from 1956 (USA & UK)

Physiological journals	Clinical science journals
Mechanisms of fat absorption	Assessment of splenectomy need in haemolytic anaemias
Anal sphincter control (cat)	
Osmoreceptors in gastric emptying	Evidence against glucostatic appetite control
	Metabolic response to gastric surgery
Aldosterone responses to dietary Na change	24-hour H^+ secretion rates in GU and DU
Acid–base status in hypothermia	Mechanisms of clearing chylomicra from plasma
Na, K and N balance in acute renal failure	Coronary blood flow $+$ O_2 consumption in hyperthyroidism
Measurement of ventilatory efficiency	Calf blood flow after revascularizing surgery
Effects of wearing high heels on leg muscle activity	Potentiation of noradrenaline pressor effect by C6
	Circulatory changes in endotoxin shock
Effects of intermittent N_2 on O_2 toxicity	WBC dynamics revealed by leucopheresis
	Causes of sickling – role of low Po_2
Fibrinolytic effect of heparin improving survival after cardiac arrest	Life span of platelets
	Experimental myocarditis from Coxsackie virus
	Fatty acids as main fuel for skeletal muscle
Factors involved in *closure* of ductus arteriosus	Lack of effect of exercise on serum cholesterol (cf. diet)
	Albumin turnover rate in man
	Albumin metabolism in nephrotic syndrome
	Protein abnormalities in agammaglobulinaemia
* Circulatory reflexes in tabes	Thyroxine-binding proteins
* Mechanisms of acclimatization to heat	Passage of steroids across the placenta
	Synovial fluid proteins in joint diseases
* Techniques of thrombin inhibition	Measurement of aldosterone in urine
	Role of aldosterone in ECF volume control
* Production and significance of electrical alternans	Competition between aminoacids for renal tubular reabsorption
* Early studies on gastric histamine receptors – clues to gastrin	Serum (K^+) and pH as evidence of K depletion
	Mechanical properties of the lungs in asthma
	Many drug studies – mercurial diuretics, anti-emetics, etc.
(* From clinical hospital departments)	Insulin hypoglycaemia symptoms due to adrenaline release

TABLE 6

The most highly relevant and original articles from 1956 (USA & UK)

Physiological journals	*Clinical science journals*
Aldosterone role in heart failure	Precipitation of liver coma by methionine
Autoregulation of cerebral blood flow	Lack of effect of glutamate in hepatic coma
Use of i.v. CO_2 to show heart structures	Familial hypoglycaemia attacks provoked by leucine
	Urinary hydroxyproline as a measure of collagen turnover
* Measurement of lung diffusing capacity	Preservation of function in a transplanted kidney
* Normal and diurnal variations in eosinophil count	Fluid and electrolyte changes in acute renal failure
* Study of thromboplastin properties	Causes of anaemia in chronic infection – (iron)
* Factors in placebo effectiveness	Causes of anaemia in cancer – (haemolysis)
* Use of noradrenaline in experimental shock	Purification of clotting factors
	Role of fibrinolytic system in bleeding disorders
* Influence of corn oil substitutes as vehicle for cholesterol feeding	Attempt to detect haemophilia carriers
	Improved blood storage techniques (nucleosides)
* Effects of experimental ureteric obstruction	Discovery of insulin-binding globulin
	Use of insulin antibodies for immunoassay
* Effects of cellulose fibre on cholesterol metabolism	Hypersensitivity to vitamin D in sarcoidosis hyper-calcaemia
	Clinical, genetic and metabolic study of congenital virilizing adrenal hyperplasia
	Dietary modification in phenylpyruvic oligophrenia
	Failure of aspirin to substitute for thyroid hormone
	Haemodynamics of general anaesthesia
	Metabolic response to burns
	Failure of hypothermia to improve recovery from bacterial infections
(* From clinical hospital departments)	Use of EDTA in lead intoxication

and clinical journals and in Table 6 I have somewhat arbitrarily selected another group of papers which seem of even higher clinical relevance. In each table I have indicated with asterisks papers published in physiological journals but coming from clinical departments. It would be pointless as well as invidious to analyse these in detail or to arrange them in any sort of order of merit, but we might note a few of the outstanding investigations. For example, an investigation into the precipitation of hepatic coma after methionine administration was reported in 1956. This provided good evidence that degradation of amino acids into toxic products by bacterial composition was responsible for the worsening of symptoms, and it reported the first preventive use of gut antibiotics. Clearly this has continued to affect the practice of clinical medicine and the management of hepatic pre-coma. In the same year we might notice that the *lack* of merit of glutamate (a substance widely used for the treatment of hepatic coma when I qualified in 1956) was finally established. We find the

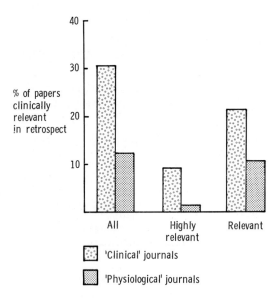

FIG. 1. (Subjective) modern relevance of papers in clinical and physiological journals in 1956.

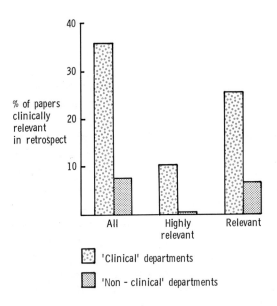

FIG. 2. (Subjective) relevance of papers from clinical and non-clinical departments in 1956

report that the hypercalcaemia of sarcoidosis had many features in common with hypervitaminosis D—a finding which we are just beginning to understand and which has had clinical repercussions in the use of steroids in the management of hypercalcaemia. The role of hyperaldosteronism in experimental heart failure was first fully documented. A planned investigation of the extent of kidney damage in dogs after different periods of complete ureteric ligation was, I think, the first study specifically designed to guide the clinician in deciding how long to wait before relieving such obstruction. (I can remember when the management of complete ureteric obstruction was extraordinarily dilatory.) The excellent physiological function of a transplanted human kidney was established by careful tests, thus laying the foundation for a modern success story of some importance. The immunoassay of insulin and identification of insulin binding proteins was also reported in 1956. The precipitation of attacks in familial hypoglycaemia by amino acids, especially leucine, was first reported. This has become the basis of a standard provocative test. The excretion of hydroxyproline as a measure of collagen turnover was first reported in this year and this has also become a widely used test.

There were also a number of honourable failures of attempts at specific therapy. For example, there was an attempt to treat experimental bacterial infection by deliberate hypothermia; there was the failure of a simple test to detect the haemophilia gene in carriers; and there was an unsuccessful attempt to substitute aspirin for thyroid hormones.

I have summarized in Fig. 1 my subjective assessment of the present-day relevance of papers published in clinical and physiological journals in 1956 under two main headings of clinical relevance. This shows a relatively small proportion of clinically relevant papers being published in the physiological journals. There is an even greater difference (Fig. 2) between the clinical relevance of papers coming from clinical departments and those from pre-clinical departments.

I feel diffident in presenting this account of a trivial investigation, the results of which will probably not surprise you at all. To be a little provocative, however, I shall end by wondering whether Lord Rothschild, who suggested that more money should be put into the support of specifically clinically relevant projects, may be to some degree supported by this sketchy retrospective study. The analysis was so tedious that I have not attempted to extend it to the present day and in any case it would be very difficult in many cases to be sure whether a paper published last year or this was likely to be influencing the practice of medicine many years hence. However, I think that the general theme which emerges—that clinical advances mostly come from clinical departments—may be worth discussion, and Dr Meyer will be reporting later in this symposium[7] his views about 'ivory towers' in French medical research. One might even be tempted to carry this line of thought still further and to take up a point rather well made by Mr Ronald Butt[8] of the *Sunday Times*, who felt that the direction of medical practice was largely governed by the personal choice of doctors and was very subject to their individual whims, and that they therefore had some public responsibility for ensuring that the direction taken by medical research was conducive to public good. In particular, perhaps we should not stimulate the public expectation for medical services which are so ludicrously extravagant that they impoverish the ordinary provision of medical care. This brief investigation suggests that by redistributing resources one may considerably influence the direction in which therapeutic advances go.

Discussion of the two preceding papers

Black: Is it quite fair to compare contributions from the basic sciences over the same period of time as for contributions from the clinical sciences?

Dickinson: There is a stage at which contributions from basic science have to reach the level of consciousness of practising doctors and then be put to experimental test. If one could devise some way of allowing for the time delay I suppose the two might come out with even honours; but the papers in the *Journal of Physiology* now seem to be getting further and further away from clinical medicine.

Fliedner: You indicated that about 30% of the clinical research papers in 1956 were highly relevant or relevant. That must mean that 70% of the money spent on clinical research is irrelevant.

Dickinson: It is probably much more than 70%. The papers I read were those accepted by journals of high quality, with fierce refereeing. Ninety per cent, or more, of the money spent on clinical research may be wasted, but this applies to research of all varieties and is inescapable: the research may be irrelevant but the money should be spent, nonetheless.

Randle: A limited journal search of this sort is perhaps less illuminating than following particular topics. One paper that I noticed was the description of insulin-binding globulin in serum by Yalow and Berson. In the *Biochemical Journal* in late 1955 (vol. 59, p. 179) Moloney and Coval published their classical paper on the induction of diabetes by injection of insulin antibodies into animals. This was certainly important in the development of radioimmunoassay, which was perhaps the biggest spin-off from the work on insulin-binding globulins. It would also be necessary to take into account work on the primary structure of insulin by Sanger, which was important in the development of insulin radioimmunoassay. The interaction was important and in this example there was an equal contribution of basic science and clinical investigation.

The 1950s were perhaps a low point in many aspects of pure physiology. There was I think a large insertion of biochemistry into physiology in the USA in that period, and many physiologists began to publish in the *Journal of Biological Chemistry* rather than the *American Journal of Physiology*. It was probably also a low period in some aspects of physiology outside of neurophysiology in the UK, so I am a little sceptical of this particular comparison.

Berliner: In 1956 the *Journal of Applied Physiology* was just getting started, and many clinical papers were being diverted to it from the *American Journal of Physiology*.

Dickinson: I agree that this influenced my findings. In England there is no journal exactly comparable to the *Journal of Applied Physiology;* many such clinical papers here would go into *Clinical Science.*

Saracci: In a sense, if 7% of papers from basic science departments are *a posteriori* classified as relevant, and 25% from clinical departments, this is what one should expect. The closer one gets to medical practice, the more one would find research papers with findings relevant to it. If controlled clinical trials were included in the survey there would surely be an even higher percentage of 'relevant' research, simply because controlled trials are generally concerned with important problems directly geared to practice. Another factor to keep in mind is the lag time between discovery and application, which is different for a basic discovery and for a finding of a more applied nature.

Dickinson: If the lag time is too long the articles will disappear almost without trace; they cease to be in the public consciousness and have to be rediscovered by somebody who starts work on the same subject again years later. I am not quite sure how to improve the analysis but I agree with your point.

Querido: Knowledge of basic science is generally applied in clinical research, and thus contributes to progress in clinical medicine. Your story reminded me of T. S. Kuhn's example concerning the date of discovery of oxygen, where he says that he can't give it because so many things contributed to that discovery.[9] For instance, the idea of doing the experiment with methionine to which you referred was generated by data and ideas which were present in the scientific community at the time. It would be interesting to pick out a few such examples and try to pursue them in that way. Theoretically the question of what would have happened if the clinical work hadn't been done is interesting. That could make the case for clinical research very strongly.

Dickinson: I agree. I am not denigrating the basic sciences at all but just trying to make an impartial investigation. There is just a slight implication that it is possible to influence the direction of research in a Rothschildian way. For example, very few people are working on chronic joint diseases, which cause an enormous amount of suffering; but if golden-egg-laying were given a larger reward more clinically valuable research would probably be done on those diseases.

Eisenberg: This study is an extremely interesting attempt in an area where the methodology is difficult. Another approach might be to look for cascade effects, using the *Science Citation Index* to trace the frequency with which a particular paper is referred to in the subsequent literature. One might look for consequences other than those immediately obvious at the time, which stimulate something even more interesting than the original results. One would also have to ask how widespread and how important the impact was. Many things that came out of one or the other investigations in 1956 may be of some limited utility in current clinical practice, but some might be massive in their impact; the importance of the discovery or its implications would have to be taken into account as well as the number of effects. A National Academy of Sciences T.R.A.C.E.S. study some time ago found that about 10% of the total funds spent on the development of the contraceptive pill went into the first papers that gave the ideas, another 10% into fundamental research exploring the ideas, and perhaps 80% into the engineering applications.

I would be loth to compare clinical science and basic science and their impact on medicine without going further than an investigation of the papers published in a single year. There are explosive consequences to ideas that become Kuhnian paradigms. It is extremely difficult to weigh that kind of impact from a given seminal idea. Although there is no disagreement about the value of supporting clinical science, Dr Campbell and Dr Dickinson failed to mention one of the greatest virtues of clinical investigation: as a physician dealing with human disease, one is in a position to see nature's experiments, which suggest possibilities the pure scientist might not have thought of so readily. This mode of analysis underestimates the potential of basic science in its ultimate contribution to clinical practice.

Hjort: One could also go about the problem the opposite way, starting from a significant improvement in clinical medicine and finding out where it came from, as in the National Academy of Sciences project you mentioned.

Berliner: Julius Comroe and Bob Dripps have just done a study like that, of the research that has yielded results relevant to advances in cardiovascular disease (*Science 192*). This study again points out that in the development of important clinical advances little of the work was originally directed towards the solution of a particular problem but turns out eventually to be useful for it.

Meyer: Dr Campbell said that clinical work had some value in improving the quality of teaching in medical schools. On the other hand Dr Dickinson mentioned that he considered himself a physiologist *manqué*. Do you think that basic teaching in medical schools could be helped by some clinicians?

Campbell: I come from a medical school which has no department of physiology. We have found that the modern specialist can teach the way his bit of the body works as well as the general-purpose physiologist. However, we run the risk that science is not fairly treated: the student can always learn to-day's stories about the way the kidney works or the lungs work but he is not likely to be interested in the scientific origin of these stories if the basic discipline of physiology is never studied in its own right.

Dickinson: I agree, but perhaps medical students should be taught more basic science by clinicians, a growing number of whom have had proper scientific training. That would also liberate departments of physiology and biochemistry from much really tedious hack work which they are expected to do. The trouble of course is that the funding of these departments depends on large numbers of medical students passing through. I can see no clear way out of this, but I certainly think there should be more basic science teaching by clinicians.

Hiatt: Sir Douglas Black suggested earlier that scientists and clinicians need to take more pains in educating their fellow citizens. This need is surely great in the United States with respect to public understanding of research. Our recent emphasis on categorical research not only leads to unreasonable expectations, but also discourages support of the gifted young scientist working at a fundamental level. If this trend continues, it could be most destructive. For example, Dr Perutz will refer to Bruce Ames, who has recently developed one of the most important assays of chemical mutagenesis, and, inferentially, of carcinogenesis. Ames's brilliant studies of the control of histidine biosynthesis began in the mid-50s. But, understandably, none of his early fundamental work was financed by cancer research funds, for neither he nor anybody else could have suspected the potential applicability of his work to cancer studies. However, this is an example of the fruits of important basic biological science soon proving to have enormous practical significance. In today's climate such basic studies by a young investigator might be difficult to fund. Simultaneously, in the United States we often hear extravagant promises about what might emerge from public support of categorical research, with the result that people expect more and more rapid 'breakthroughs', which cannot, of course, keep pace. It would be profitable if we considered how to help the public to understand that what will be the practical significance of fundamental research cannot be predicted in advance. Of course, we must also support applied research, but it is fruitless to seek applications prematurely.

Dr Dickinson did not suggest that 'relevance' should be the sole determinant of how money should be allocated for research. Yet people do look to us for some kind of formula for determining how much of our resources should be dedicated to fundamental and how much to applied research.

Dickinson: I am not sure, Dr Hiatt, whether we shouldn't consider some change in the allocation of resources. You mentioned the millions of dollars spent on cancer research. Two notable advances in the active therapy of cancer stem, at least in the first step back, from clinicians. One is the treatment of hormone-dependent cancer by oophorectomy and adrenalectomy. The other is the special technique of treating chorionepithelioma by using established drugs titrated by the chemical marker. A few of those dollars might perhaps have been better spent by clinicians in contact with cancer patients rather than by people working in laboratories on rats and mice.

Eisenberg: Some countries may not have to invest very much in basic research because they can take advantage of what goes on elsewhere. The Chinese, for example, have been notably pragmatic in synthesizing and copying the drugs that have come from the West. If we were to follow their example in doing very little fundamental investigation it would be a tragic loss for them as well as us.

Bull: I agree with Dr Campbell that the borderline between practice and research is very tenuous. I would like to go further and say that to do clinical research properly, one has also to provide a practical service. First, a clinician has to carry out some service to remain competent clinically. Secondly, often the most exciting and interesting things in disease derive from the exception rather than the rule, and to get the exceptional patients a fairly large number is needed. Therefore one has to provide some service that others do not, so that enough patients are referred.

In 1955 I investigated a number of journals in which people working in clinical departments in England would be expected to publish. I wrote to the departmental heads and found out the number of beds and the number of staff in those hospitals, then plotted the figures against the number of publications per department. There was a linear regression giving a correlation coefficient of above 0.9 between them. This means that 80% of the research output as measured by publication was predictable from the staffing. There must be a certain minimum number of staff before there is any research. In those days the figure was eight doctors per hundred beds. Then publications went up linearly.

Woodruff: Your conclusions, Dr Dickinson, depend a bit on the definition of clinical science. At first I thought you meant that component of clinical research which has nothing to do with treatment and is concerned only with investigation. But if advances in therapeutics, applied pharmacology and so on are included one would have to read a different set of journals and one would certainly come up with a different set of conclusions. For example it is inconceivable that Fleming's work on *Penicillium notatum* would have been published in the *Journal of Physiology*, and it seems equally inconceivable that Florey and Chain would have published their work in the *Journal of Clinical Investigation*. Obviously it would be a Herculean task to analyse all the relevant journals, but I don't think the kind of answer you find can be very field-related. It would be a little unfortunate if the term clinical science, which is a term we should treasure, had removed from it any component of advances in therapeutics.

Gelzer: You were discussing the value of clinical science but you hardly mentioned the word 'patient', Dr Dickinson. Did you assess the relevance of clinical science in terms of utility to the doctor, or to science only, or did you also take utility to the patient into consideration? Was your assessment of utility based on your own subjective feeling, or on objective criteria such as shorter stays in hospital or greater comfort for the sick?

Dickinson: It was more a gut feeling as a general physician asking what difference something made to one's management of a patient and to a patient's expectation of getting better quickly. It was very vague.

What Dr Bull said about the necessity of research and progress reminds me that Flexner in his autobiography has a marvellous definition of a profession as an activity in which practice and progress are closely interwoven and react upon each other.[10] One can't imagine medicine continuing to exist as a profession unless medical progress is going on.

Dornhorst: Your presentation has effectively defended clinical science from the charge of triviality, Dr Dickinson. That list of subjects has become part of the intellectual furniture of practising clinicians. But it would be a mistake to draw conclusions from those data about which journals to read or where to spend research funds.

Perutz: I was impressed by the usefulness of the clinical research you listed for 1956, Dr Dickinson. But I must spring to the defence of non-clinical research. We should measure not just the number of studies but also their importance. In the nature of things the number of fundamentally important discoveries in any one year is few, but even a single one may become the source of great advances in clinical and other sciences. I remember 1956 as the year when Ingram demonstrated that sickle cell anaemia is due to the replacement of a single amino acid residue in haemoglobin.[11,12] That established the chemical basis for our understanding of inherited diseases, and has helped in their diagnosis and in the rationalization of their treatment. Perhaps not as much as one million dollars was spent on molecular biology in the world in that year, yet it produced that one gem.

Beeson: The mention of haemoglobin illustrates something that concerns me about clinical research. We clinicians have become pretty good at applying basic sciences to clinical problems but rarely can we do the best possible job. We have tended to grow apart from the basic scientists and currently have little opportunity for communication with them. Yet, as has been pointed out, we have the unique advantage of observing 'experiments of nature', which provide great leads. The haemoglobin story really began with a train ride, when Bill Castle and Linus Pauling were travelling to a committee meeting in Denver. Castle described to Pauling this peculiar disorder (sickle cell anaemia) in which the red cells take on an odd form at times. They agreed that there must be something wrong with the haemoglobin. This was a kind of interdisciplinary communication that I think we are missing.

Any clinician with a special interest in a group of diseases could probably point out some surprisingly neglected areas. From my own special interest in infection, I am intrigued by the fact that common microbial infections by extracellular parasites such as *E. coli* or *Pneumococcus* have preferences for certain organs and they don't infect other organs. No one ever heard of a pneumococcal infection of the kidney, and one rarely hears of an *E. coli* infection of the lung. There must be something in the biochemical milieu of these organs that will support infection with certain extracellular pathogens and not with others. Here is a surprisingly neglected area of study; I don't think the average clinician has the ability to attack a problem like that. It is too bad that we are not passing such challenges on to the Perutzes of this world.

Phillips: The communication problem is perhaps the most challenging aspect of the somewhat false dichotomy between basic and clinical research. It is often surprisingly difficult to get basic scientists and clinical scientists together, but when they do get together it is often very fruitful. In the US one finds people doing protein chemistry in a back room and looking after patients in the front room, but in the UK that doesn't happen so often.

Dickinson: One vehicle for the collaboration between preclinical or basic sciences and clinical departments ought to be the common room. It is a pity that most common rooms for preclinical and clinical people are entirely separate in the UK. The possibilities of proper collaboration in clinical and basic science were nicely illustrated by my last experience in this room, at the Ciba Foundation Symposium on Lung Liquids.[12a] The combination of basic scientists and clinicians was an immensely productive exercise from which we all derived new ideas. I can't imagine that either the basic scientists or the clinicians felt disappointed. Perhaps we need to force more mixing, both by simple geographical arrangements of common rooms and by conferences especially planned to mix basic and clinical scientists.

Eisenberg: Mention has been made of the difficult ethical problems in doing research. What should be equally emphasized are the ethical problems of not doing research. To some extent, the preoccupation with patients' rights and the hazards of research leads to the fact being overlooked that it is only by research that the public can be protected from the hazards of many conventional medical procedures. Discussion of the ethics of research must include a comprehensive review of what happens when there is no research. What are the consequences of being so preoccupied with the risks that go with something experimental that one overlooks entirely the risks that go with conventional procedures that have only the sanction of time and tradition to support them? In clinical science, the internist and the pharmacologist have to have their procedures approved by hospital committees or government regulations before investigations can be undertaken. Our surgical colleagues could also benefit from such controls. Once a procedure that seems to be effective has been introduced it becomes extremely difficult to set up a controlled clinical trial, because the impression is widespread that something of value is being withheld. I would argue that it is unethical *not* to do research; that is one of the aspects of clinical science that should be made clear to the public.

Owen: Dr Campbell (p. 45) mentioned the rigorous way in which the ethics of clinical research are now controlled all over the world. We now have the Tokyo revision[13] of the Declaration of Helsinki as well as the Medical Research Council's own statement on the ethics of experimentation in human subjects.[14] In the United Kingdom, all clinical research investigations require the prior approval of a local ethical committee; and similar arrangements apply in most other countries. We have all that in clinical research, yet there is a dramatic contrast with the lack of any systematic ethical audit or surveillance of clinical practice. In England one can't legally make a venous puncture for research purposes in a child under the age of consent, but any procedure however heroic and however unestablished is permissible if the parents can be persuaded of its possible diagnostic or therapeutic value. This contrast has developed during the last twenty-five years and is now very obvious.

Campbell: I am more worried about the harm done by investigations and treatments that clinicians use, and for which there is little evidence of benefit, than I am about the conduct of research by sound clinical scientists.

I would like to suggest that we need to examine what we mean by science. I don't necessarily think of science and research as the same thing. Dr Eisenberg used the word science to mean 'hard' subjects like physics and chemistry and so on, whereas I think science consists of a corpus of refutable but not yet refuted ideas, not confined to physics and chemistry.

That leads me on to an educational point. There is the danger that science is seen by the medical student as just a corpus of the so-called hard basic sciences, whereas science is an attitude of mind. There is a false antithesis between science and the humanities and a false association between science and technology. I would say that the problem in medicine is too much technology and not enough science, rather than the other way round. Many scientists regard the intuitive and imaginative component of science, rather than the practical importance of the problems it tackles, as the highest achievement. If this is so, it is going to be difficult to get scientists who value themselves according to the originality of their ideas to tackle important research problems which call for the grammar of science but don't have the intellectually imaginative excitement of science. I am not trying to be élitist, but just making a point which I think explains some of the difficulties we will have in promoting research on issues which require scientific good manners but are not truly scientific matters.

References

[1] CAMPBELL, E. J. M. (1976) Clinical science, in this volume, pp. 41-52
[2] *American Journal of Physiology* (1956) All papers in vols. 184-187
[3] *Journal of Physiology (London) (1956)* All papers in vols. 131-134
[4] *Journal of Clinical Investigation* (1956) All papers in vol. 44
[5] *Clinical Science* (1956) All papers in vol. 15
[6] MEDAWAR, P. B. (1967) *The Art of the Soluble*, Methuen, Londen
[7] MEYER, P. (1976) French medical research. the risk of 'demedicalization', in this volume, pp. 137-145
[8] BUTT, R. (1974) The needs of patients. *Proceedings of the Royal Society of Medicine 67*, 1297-1300
[9] KUHN, T. S. (1970) *The Structure of Scientific Revolution*, 2nd edn., University of Chicago Press, Chicago
[10] FLEXNER, A. (1940) *I Remember*, Simon & Schuster, New York
[11] INGRAM, V. M. (1956) A specific chemical difference between the globins of normal human and sickle-cell anaemia haemoglobin. *Nature (London) 178*, 792-794
[12] INGRAM, V. M. (1957) Gene mutations in human haemoglobin: the chemical difference be-ween normal and sickle cell haemoglobin. *Nature (London) 180*, 326-328
[12a] CIBA FOUNDATION (1976) *Lung Liquids (Ciba Found. Symp. 38)*, Elsevier/Excerpta Medica/North-Holland, Amsterdam
[13] World Medical Association (1975) *Declaration of Helsinki, 1964*, as revised by the 29th World Medical Assembly, Tokyo, Japan; World Medical Association, Fermey-Voltaire
[14] Medical Research Council (1963) *Report of the Medical Research Council 1962-1963*, pp. 21-25, Medical Research Council, London

The assessment of efficacy, toxicity and quality of care in long-term drug treatment

C. T. DOLLERY

Dept of Clinical Pharmacology, Royal Postgraduate Medical School, London

Abstract Drug studies in man are usually divided into four phases. The first phase is to establish that the drug has a pharmacological action in man and in which dose range it occurs. The second phase is a study of the therapeutic effect of the drug in small numbers of closely observed patients. The third phase consists of large-scale studies which may involve hundreds or thousands of patients; such studies are designed to accumulate less detailed information about efficacy and to provide information about low frequency toxic events. At the end of this stage the drug is submitted to a regulatory body for a license to market it.

Information derived from these studies usually has several important deficiencies. There is unlikely to be much evidence about the efficacy of the drug in relation to that of other substances used to treat the same condition. The carefully regulated conditions of the clinical trial may bear little relationship to the way the drug will be used in practice. Most important, the evidence obtained on efficacy may relate chiefly to the pharmacological action of the drug, e.g. in lowering blood pressure or blood sugar, or reducing inflammation, and may not bear directly upon therapeutic outcome. For these reasons much attention is being focused on monitoring of the way drugs are used after marketing. To provide evidence of therapeutic efficacy may require studies of such large scale and high cost that they are beyond the reach of individual pharmaceutical companies and will require national or international action. Monitoring of the way drugs are used inevitably means studying not just the performance of the drug but also of the doctors who prescribe it. Studies that have been made of the quality of care of patients treated with anti-hypertensive drugs and those requiring anticoagulants are not reassuring concerning the general level of such quality.

The influence of basic biomedical research on medical practice can be seen more clearly in the field of drug therapy than in any other aspect of medicine. Modern therapeutics has been created by basic and clinical research. The discovery of the antibacterial activity of the red dye, Prontosil, in the 1930s, was the starting point for an invaluable series of drugs descended from the sulphonamides, and for an even more important concept, chemical manipulation of the internal environment of man to fight disease. The almost miraculous quality of some of the discoveries is easily forgotten but it would be difficult to contemplate our modern civilized western world without its medicines. My purpose in this paper is not to relive some of the victories in the march of pharmacology but to consider research in pharmacology and therapeutics as a model of many of the problems and some of the solutions to the questions posed by the title of this symposium.

Pharmacology and therapeutics cover the entire spectrum from the most basic spatial concepts in chemistry to the delivery of medical care by the practitioner when the drug synthesized by the chemist has become a part of the standard armamentarium of therapeutics. In the initial stages of the therapeutic revolution a highly productive chaos reigned and, considering how powerful the chemical entities were that were administered to man, disasters were surprisingly few.

When a new drug was synthesized, it was usually derived from a natural product or a known active structure. (This activity is now referred to disparagingly as molecular roulette and is held to be undesirable, yet many of the drugs we now use were arrived at by this means, and it is more rational than the hand of chance which has also played a significant part.) The new structure was then examined for chemical purity and tested in animal preparations to see what pharmacological activity it might possess. If it proved to be active, the median lethal dose, the LD_{50}, would be measured and some limited chronic dosing studies would be done. Then an interested clinician had to be found who would try the drug out on a patient, with or without his or her knowledge and consent. If the clinician was careful, the hazards were not large, and if the drug looked promising it would not be long before it was on the market and could be prescribed by anyone. Unfortunately, there were catastrophes and of these thalidomide had more impact than any other because of the particular horror of children being born deformed after a drug had been prescribed for trivial symptoms. In most countries regulatory bodies for drugs have been created to reconcile the conflicting interests of patients, investigators, practitioners and manufacturers. The longest-established of these bodies is the Food and Drug Administration in the USA, and in the discussion that follows I shall use their terminology, which divides drug investigations into four phases.

I shall take it as axiomatic that new drugs are still needed to treat many human diseases and that both new and old drugs must be used effectively to treat those who may benefit from them.

OBJECTIVES OF DIFFERENT PHASES OF DRUG ADMINISTRATION IN MAN

The objectives of different phases of drug investigation vary greatly and it is essential to consider them individually. I do not intend to cover the preclinical phase, but simply to say that it is the indispensable progenitor of what follows.

Phase I

The question asked in Phase I is straightforward: 'Is there a pharmacological action in man that might be useful in therapy?'

The parties concerned are the innovators, the chemists, pharmacologists, toxicologists and medical practitioners in industry, and the clinical pharmacologists, usually working in academic centres. Often the research is carried out on normal volunteers and these individuals are quite frequently the investigators themselves and their immediate colleagues. The aims of the research, although usually in the long term commercial, are almost entirely expressed in rigorous scientific terms. The standards of experimental design and conduct are usually fairly high and have risen in the last decade.

Often the work will require skilful collaboration between clinical pharmacologists who can measure drug effects and biochemical pharmacologists who seek explanations for these effects in terms of the fate of the drug in the human body. If a Phase I study of a drug is carried out in normal volunteers it does not involve any outside regulatory body, although the Ethics Committee of the institution must give its consent. Most investigators in this field are of the opinion that it would be sensible to take more new chemical entities to Phase I so that the best choice can be made between different structures that are candidate drugs. Obviously I have a professional interest to defend in this regard, but this opinion is held by people other than those directly involved.

Phase II

The question to be answered in the Phase II trial is once again clearcut; it is 'Is the pharmacological action demonstrated in Phase I useful in therapy?' The simplicity of Phase I is lost in Phase II because the number of parties involved increases and their interests are not identical. A drug regulatory body, in the UK the Committee on Safety of Medicines, which advises the licensing authority (the Department of Health and Social Security) and issues a Clinical Trial Certificate, must give its consent. This will lead to delay, which may or may not be in the public interest. If the drug is a valuable innovation the delay is harmful; if it proves of little value or is toxic the delay may mean that un-pleasant discovery being made on the citizens of another land with consequent credit to whoever caused the delay. At this stage the main issue considered by the Committee on Safety of Medicines is the safety of the drug and, to a lesser extent, the qualifications of the investigator. The public interest is not brought in to any great extent because, until the activity of the drug is known, the public interest cannot be ascertained.

Patients are involved, as they may be in Phase I, with some types of drugs. In the early days of treatment when there were few effective drugs the interests of patients were often well served if they participated in clinical trials. They were the first to receive the new wonder drug. Nowadays the position is cloudier because a more likely outcome is that the patient in a trial may receive a medicine that is no more effective, and possibly less effective, than a standard one. It is in the public interest that the trial should be done, but it is not so evidently in the individual's interest. This is a dilemma that will need more consid-eration in the future, and Ethics Committees are possibly not a full safeguard. One helpful development would be a generous no-fault insurance for patients taking part in Phase II studies, to compensate them against non-negligent mishaps.

Phase III

In Phase III the horizon widens again, for the intention is to expand the numbers included in the Phase II trial so that more precise evidence of efficacy over a longer period of time can be obtained, and so that the importance of relatively low frequency toxic events can be evaluated. Serious toxicity, such as the oculocutaneous syndrome with practolol, may cause a drug to be severely restricted or withdrawn if it occurs as often as once per thousand patients treated. There may be little likelihood that a Phase III clinical trial can detect such a low frequency event but it ought at least to detect something that occurs once in every hundred patients treated.

As Phase III trials use much larger numbers of patients it is inevitable that the skill of the investigators will be less and their facilities fewer than in the earlier part of the study. In some respects it is acceptable that this should be so because it is closer to the conditions of practice. Unfortunately the standard of record-keeping is often lower as well, so that the quality of evidence is not adequate for drawing firm conclusions. In fact it is a basic dilemma of research at this stage as to how useful data can be collected without drastically altering the normal pattern of medical practice.

It is very important that Phase III trials should include comparative obser-vations against whatever regimen is the standard one for the disease under study. Pharmaceutical companies with highly original products are only too keen to compare them with existing remedies, but the enthusiasm is less if the new product bears a marked resemblance to an existing one. I believe it is in the public interest that regulatory authorities should insist on such comparative evidence before they issue a product licence permitting general sale at public expense. Unfortunately the drafting of the Medicines Act does not allow the Committee on Safety of Medicines to take relative efficiency into account except where this has a relevance to safety. I consider that it would be a reasonable requirement that for drugs that are to be provided free under the National Health Service it should be demonstrated that they are no less effective than drugs already available, and preferably that there are circumstances in which they are better. However, it must be admitted that it is often difficult to reach such a decision on the evidence available at the time of marketing. For the present I would suggest that the National Health Service might decline to pay for drugs that are significantly less effective than standard ones, and that a drug should be required to have evidence that it is not significantly less effective before it is accepted by the NHS.

Product licence

At the conclusion of the Phase III trials a marketing submission is made to the Committee on Safety of Medicines, which gives detailed consideration to the efficacy, safety and clinical indications for the drug, as well as to technical matters like stability, purity, etc. The Committee clearly represents both public and professional interests but, in some ways, it represents the latter more than the former. When I was a member of the Committee I sometimes felt that a voice of the public should have said just before every decision about a product licence 'Is it in the public interest that this drug should be available on prescription?' In many instances the answer might have been neutral even if it had not been negative.

The issue of a product licence is a fundamental stage in drug development because there must be positive evidence of a harmful effect before it is likely to be cancelled.

Phase IV

The end of Phase III clinical trials and the granting of a product licence which permits the drug to be marketed have all too often marked the end of the involvement of research workers. The use of the drug in the ordinary practice of medicine was left to the market place, the collective opinion of doctors pushed and pulled by the retail men and the brightly coloured advertisements in the post and journals. I do not entirely despise the judgement of the market place concerning the relative worth of one drug against another of a similar type, but I find it surprising that so little attention has been paid to the way drugs are used in practice as compared to the regulated environment of the clinical trial. Nothing so clearly demarcates the division between biomedical research and health services research as the transition from clinical trial certificate to product licence.

Until very recently there have been two main concerns about this stage of investigation, often now dignified by the title 'Phase IV'. The first arose directly from thalidomide and it led to the organization of effective adverse reaction warning systems. The UK has been more successful than most other countries in establishing a central reporting system for collecting and analysing spontaneous reports from doctors on the adverse effects of medicines they have prescribed. It was data of this sort that led to the recommendation that the oestrogen content of the contraceptive pill should be reduced to diminish the risk of thromboembolism. Obviously, reporting of adverse reactions is highly important, but a highly distorted view of the world of therapeutics is obtained by looking at it solely through the eyes of an expert on adverse drug reactions. Without detailed knowledge of benefit, it is hard to assess the significance of the darker side of the coin.

The second concern has been with cost. In many countries the main cost of drugs falls on a government agency—in the UK the National Health Service. Medicines have taken about 10% of the cost of the NHS throughout its history. As the service was founded at a time of unprecedented advance in therapeutics the stability of this percentage seems surprising. Governments are concerned to save expenditure especially when the payment is to a third party, not a direct employee. The NHS uses various devices such as histograms illustrating relative costs to try and persuade doctors to prescribe more economically. To set against these concerns about adverse effects and cost there are few data save national mortality figures from which to judge whether the risks and expenditure are justified. What little is known about the effectiveness of medicines in general use is not entirely reassuring. Four examples will serve to illustrate some of the problems.

Tricyclic antidepressants are effective in relieving severe depression in most patients, but their full effect takes about three weeks to develop. Unfortunately, side effects such as dry mouth, blurred vision and difficulty in emptying the bladder begin almost at once. Johnson followed up depressed patients diagnosed by general practitioners and found that only 72% who might have benefited from tricyclic antidepressants received them, and 59% of these had ceased to take the drug within three weeks.[1] Thus, only about 29% received what is usually regarded as optimal treatment.

Many elderly patients who suffer lower limb fractures develop deep vein thromboses and pulmonary emboli. Sevitt and Gallagher demonstrated that prophylactic use of anticoagulants considerably reduced mortality and almost abolished death from pulmonary emboli.[2] Recently Morris and Mitchell[3] conducted a postal survey on the use of prophylactic anticoagulants in such patients by British orthopaedic surgeons. They received replies from 411 surgeons (64% response), and of these only 3% routinely used anticoagulants in elderly patients with hip fractures.

Antihypertensive drugs have been shown to greatly prolong life in patients with malignant hypertension.[4] A recent study based on scrutiny of case notes of patients who died in Greater London and whose death certificates mentioned malignant hypertension revealed some interesting aspects of their care. All those who died whose blood pressure could be ascertained had inadequate control of blood pressure before death, and in some cases the pressure had scarcely been controlled at all for years. Less than a quarter of the general practice notes had a blood pressure recorded in them for visits after the diagnosis of malignant hypertension had been made.[5]

All these are examples of under-use of drugs, but the contrary situation is also commonplace. Cochrane studied the use of vitamin B_{12} in Wales and concluded that about ten times as much was being used as was likely to be needed to treat patients with pernicious anaemia and malabsorption syndromes.[6]

A further aspect of Phase IV studies that is at last receiving attention is the efficacy of drugs in long-term use. Many drugs have been introduced into therapy on the assumption that their pharmacological action was likely to be beneficial because they restored some deranged biochemical factor towards normal. When the biochemical abnormality is the disease, as in vitamin or hormone deficiencies, this assumption is usually justified but in other circumstances caution is needed. Drugs that lower blood lipids or blood sugar have been widely used because it was assumed that they would thereby prevent or minimize the vascular complications of hyperlipidaemias and diabetes. The results of clinical trials such as the University Group Diabetes Program and the Coronary Drug Project[7, 8] which failed to demonstrate benefit and even— in the Diabetes Program—suggested harm, illustrate the frailty of such assumptions. It is also worth noting that these trials were mounted by government agencies and not by the pharmaceutical houses that developed the products under study. The cost of such long-term trials is so high and the work makes so many demands on skilled personnel that it is unlikely that a single pharmaceutical company would have the money or the personnel to arrange such a study. Work of this kind could be a fruitful area for international collaboration in medical research if the funding and administrative problems could be solved.

CONCLUSIONS

Basic and clinical research created modern therapeutics, the most important single achievement of medicine. Creativity in this field is by no means at an end. Immunology, oncology and central nervous system pharmacology are ripe for major therapeutic advances. Yet the carry-through of research into practice has been deficient. Some drugs are prescribed excessively and others less often than they should be. Many are used skilfully, but some of the most important drugs require more skill, if they are to be used to best advantage, than most prescribers seem to possess.

None of the problems at the applied end will be solved by stifling research at the basic biomedical end. I have little patience with some of my colleagues in epidemiology and sociology who argue that the community would benefit from a major diversion of resources from the basic to the applied end. But the epidemiologists and the sociologists have powerful arguments for some change of emphasis. As I have just said, ten times as much vitamin B_{12} is prescribed as is needed to treat pernicious anaemia, and only 3% of orthopaedic surgeons use prophylactic anticoagulants in the elderly with hip fractures, although the value of such treatment has been proved.

It is high time that the interest of the medical profession in Phase IV studies of drugs shifted away from a near-total preoccupation with adverse effects and towards the efficacy of the drugs being used and ways of improving the mode of use to make them more effective. In some instances this will mean using less drugs and in others more, and in many cases it will mean using them with greater care and discrimination. These problems are a proper subject for research, but it is to be hoped that this will not be purely descriptive but will test by randomized controlled trials better ways of providing information and utilizing drugs. The present trial of treatment in mild hypertension which is being organized by the Medical Research Council is one example of what ought to be done. A substantial effort is also needed to improve the delivery of health care with drugs and this will require research of a new type. Collecting evidence of poor quality work is only the first step. Intervention is needed to test procedures that may improve the way drugs are used routinely. Such research must look closely at general practice because 90% of the prescriptions of the NHS are written by general practitioners. The willingness of the profession to permit scrutiny of their work and to devise methods of measuring the effective-ness of drugs prescribed in a general practice will both pose major challenges.

I have argued elsewhere[9] that organized audit of health care by professional groups must become an established part of medical practice, and this may be supplemented by special studies of particular problems such as the confidential enquiry into maternal mortality. The activities of such audit groups will themselves require evaluation but the case for action of some kind seems strong enough already without the need for a great deal more discussion.

I end by returning to the therapeutic spectrum with which I began. Just as red and blue are essential components of the white light of a real spectrum, so the basic biomedical side and the applied side of pharmacological research are essential to one another. The research community needs to look at the whole spectrum and be funded to do so. It cannot be left to the pharmaceutical industry alone to decide how drugs shall be promoted and used. The battle of Phase IV, the way drugs are used in practice, must be joined.

Discussion

Black: You rightly said that drug therapy is an area in which biomedical and health services research tend to merge. Dr Dollery. The two themes of this conference merge in relation to drug therapy, which is also important in medical education.

Owen: A fundamental question here is, to what extent do the results of medical research influence medical practice? Where there is a glaring example of clear-cut research being ignored in practice, as the orthopaedic surgeons did in your example, is it worth doing the research? Should the Department of Health and Social Security or the Medical Research Council spend some millions of pounds on trials of antihypertensive drugs in mild to moderate hypertension when it seems unlikely that, whatever the results, medical practice will be significantly influenced?

Dollery: The anticoagulants may be a special case. About eight or ten years ago the main question was about their use in arterial disease, where any benefit was clearly small. The vituperative arguments were, properly, won by those who opposed their use. Anticoagulants were therefore felt to be not much good, but no distinction was made between arterial and venous disease, though it was always clear that these drugs are beneficial in thromboembolic disease.

In the MRC trial of mild to moderate hypertension 87% of patients took 75% or more of their medicines. That is really not bad, though only 54% of them took 90% or more. Of course it may well be that outside a trial context these patients would not take the drugs so reliably. But as some 10% of the population of the UK are hypertensive it is important to know whether treatment benefits them. If it does, the next question will be whether they can be persuaded to take their medicine, but by then we will know whether it is worth getting them to do so. If it is not, we should be able to save the country a lot of money, by persuading doctors not to use drugs that are not worth while. On the other hand, if a drug is beneficial, then maybe we will have to look for another drug that is even more effective, with a longer duration of action—the one-shot treatment that I mentioned earlier (p. 38).

Woodruff: If a patient gets a carcinoma of the pancreas or ruptures his aortic aneurysm it is thought of as a kind of act of God, but if he dies after an operation for such conditions it is often felt to be due to the incompetence of the surgeon. That is another reason why people sometimes hesitate to apply something new.

Owen: Dr Dollery said there were sins of commission as well as omission. Many would feel that waiting lists for adenotonsillectomy were still unnecessarily long.

Burgen: I think we are still in the aftermath of the time when the emphasis of clinical medicine was on diagnosis and much treatment was surgical. The attention given to non-surgical therapeutic measures then was minimal.

We still have a large generation of doctors who trained under those conditions, and also a large generation of doctors who train doctors under those conditions. A really radical reappraisal is needed. We all accept that the object of medicine is to treat patients and get them better, and that therefore treatment ought to be the most important thing in medical schools and in hospitals. Quite contrary to this, the spread of clinical pharmacology has been slow in the UK. There are still schools without either major teaching officers or good departments. I don't think there is a single non-teaching hospital with a clinical pharmacologist in it. The amount of follow-up information that general practitioners and other doctors receive about the proper use of drugs is minimal, yet this is perhaps where one of the biggest pay-offs in medical practice could come. A tremendous programme of re-education is needed, and the most important is probably re-education for medical teachers.

Pickering: I agree strongly with what Dr Dollery said. I wish I had the same confidence as he has in medical education. Those depressing results about anticoagulants and fractures of the hip reflect the attitude of mind of orthopaedic surgeons, an attitude which they developed when they were medical students about thirty years ago, when the value of scientific evidence was not appreciated by medical students. I am doing a survey of medical education now and I regret to say that the value of scientific evidence is still not appreciated by the medical student, nor indeed do his teachers mind whether it is appreciated.

The student is never examined on scientific method. Now it is all multiple choice questions. One group of students said they had done nothing but put ticks in little squares on paper since the age of sixteen, so how were they expected to write decent English? The rising generation is not going to be any better than the old one.

Marinker: There are all sorts of problems about the use of drugs in practice, that is in 'Phase IV'. In general practice, where most drugs are prescribed, diagnosis is usually at the symptomatic not the causal level. Johnson's paper on patients taking tricyclic antidepressants illustrates the difficulties well.[1] I was not nearly so depressed as you about that paper, Dr Dollery. A diagnosis of clinical depression carries a strong subjective element on the part of the doctor. So what the paper reflects is a difference between the subjective impressions of the psychiatrist (Johnson) and those of the general practitioners who made the diagnoses. The effect of tricyclic drugs does not begin until between about ten days and three weeks. In that lag period the patient experiences only the bad effects of the drugs. Tricyclic antidepressants anyway are not as specific in their actions as, for example, the antibiotics are for a sensitive microorganism. There are an enormous number of variables. The use of psychotropic drugs in general practice seems quite irrational. This perhaps reflects the fact that it is difficult, using the present diagnostic frameworks, for a doctor to ascribe a disease to a patient who presents with an illness that the doctor can't explain. The doctor translates the illness into a psychiatric disease, either depression or anxiety, for which there is a whole library of responses.

In general practice the commonest presenting symptom is a sore throat, but there is no defined body of knowledge that tells the general practitioner whether the best thing to prescribe is penicillin.

Dornhorst: I agree with Sir Arnold Burgen that we are in a particular historical phase of development where the attitude to drugs is changing. It has indeed already changed in teaching centres, but we still have the inevitable lag before this is effective in practice. One major change should be in the traditional view that drugs are indicated by diseases, and that when the clinician has given the drug after making the diagnosis he has done all he needs to do. That view was fine when it was a question of whether to give valerian or bromide and so on, because then it did not really matter. Nowadays we have a wide array of potent drugs which can dramatically affect the working of the body. Drugs must now be regarded as things which will alter the physiology of the body— beneficially, it is hoped, but perhaps harmfully. The low numbers of people taking their antihypertensive drugs is perhaps shocking but it is not surprising. Any consultant who has tried to send hypertensive patients back to their general practitioners in a well-controlled state knows that the chances of the patients continuing to be well controlled is quite low. This may stem from the attitude that if the drug is given that is the end of it and there is no need to measure the blood pressure again. One also finds that when the blood pressure is measured again and is normal, the drug is then stopped. This attitude must change. Serious teaching about clinical pharmacology has lagged but it is now improving. It will take time before this works its way out into practice.

Owen: I agree. Nevertheless it really proves that there is something missing from the title of this symposium. The interface is not between medical research and medical practice but between medical research and medical education, which then influences practice.

Dornhorst: That includes postgraduate education, of course, but the main thing is the undergraduate education. It is the fundamental attitude that matters.

Campbell: The two examples, one of hypertension and one of anticoagulants, illustrate two different problems. In Hamilton, Ontario, where I work, orthopaedic surgeons would now be liable to criticism if they did not use anticoagulants. This is because of the audit in hospitals. I think this should be the way of the future. The surgeon takes the strategic decision that the patient should receive antiagulant treatment but other people who are experts at anticoagulation administer the drugs. The standard of management has greatly improved.

Secondly, to turn to the treatment of hypertension, this is a specific example of a problem affecting several other health matters. That is, how do we decide that somebody be allowed to do anything to large numbers of people in society? It is almost a 'Catch 22' situation: we don't know whether it is the right decision until we have taken the decision; we would rather not take the decision until we have the information; and we won't have the information until we have taken the decision! There is a gap in our methodology between the specific study of a particular problem like the effect of a drug in a restricted population —such as people with a raised blood pressure—and the techniques with a low signal-to-noise ratio such as the census or survey. It seems to me that we haven't really got a way of coping with problems like introducing new drugs, particularly drugs that are taken widely for minor symptoms. We cannot take a decision and see its consequences before making the decision irrevocable. Perhaps modern survey techniques might be able to bridge this gap and lessen the need for expensive *ad hoc* studies such as the hypertension study referred to.

Dollery: We should carry out organized clinical trials in Phase IV. The Coronary Drug Project[8] and the MRC trials are examples of this being done. But some people in the MRC seem to be reacting against the large sums of money these trials cost. In my opinion they are wrong: the questions the trials are designed to answer are of great importance.

Education, although essential, is not enough. I have argued elsewhere[9] that an organized audit of health care is needed. Whether that would be provided on an area, district, regional or national basis I don't know, but it would have to be professional, with doctors auditing doctors. For general practice, where about 90 % of all drugs used in the UK are prescribed, the only way of influencing the situation is by some kind of auditing procedure. Even if a hospital has no official auditing procedure, a great deal of auditing goes on, simply because people's decisions are overlooked by many other people, who criticize them openly or otherwise. General practice has nothing like that, but there is a necessity to introduce it. It could be done by selecting particular well-defined problems, such as the confidential enquiry into maternal mortality, or it could be done more generally, for example by audit of hospital emergency services. Probably both will have to be done.

Marinker: Audit as a method of postgraduate education for general practitioners is the best way forward. There has to be some audit of, for example, prescribing as the management of hypertension in the practice population. We are looking at this in Leicester now. Until there is self-criticism in general practice, all the research in the world will be ignored.

Campbell: I believe strongly that medical students should learn about science, not just learn the stories of science. Doctors should know the principles of drug use. But that is not necessarily the way to tackle the problem of ensuring that a defined group of patients in a hospital is adequately treated with anticoagulants. That is a separate issue. I would like to think that the profession can judge the evidence but then accepts that implementation of the goal of anticoagulation is too complicated for the orthopaedic surgeon. I agree with the need for education and I agree with the therapeutic aim, but I don't think education is the tactical means of achieving the therapeutic end.

Black: One would not want orthopaedic surgeons to determine the precise anticoagulant regimen, but it is a matter of taking a clinical decision to have it done.

Fliedner: In the United Kingdom you can base many therapeutic recommendations on the results of MRC trials. In Germany, we do not have such controlled trials. Before anybody can be educated, follow-up studies are needed on the right procedures for the management of certain diseases. We have just tackled a particular example, hypertension, but there must be hundreds of diseases for which there is no established method of management. And there is no factual evidence on whether Dr A has better success with his treatment than Dr B. Unless we have follow-up statistics on the various types of management there is little we can teach students that will help their performance as general practitioners. Near a medical school there is always the possibility of better treatment than further out in the country. Therefore a patient might live or die depending on the distance he lives from a particular medical school.

Who is going to make decisions about clinical science and its ethical and social implications? Here we have dealt with fairly simple examples of how things can be improved. But clinical science provides many modes of treatment, apart from drugs. If some of these methods are used for *all* patients with certain diseases, no country could afford to pay the cost. For example, if everybody who in principle would benefit from an artificial pancreas for diabetes were given one, where would the money come from? And which organizations are thinking about the social and ethical implications of clinical research? Where is the organization that thinks about areas that are not fashionable in clinical science but are important for the health of the population?

Black: The MRC and the DHSS share those responsibilities in the UK.

Bull: When a new drug is introduced which is clearly effective it is immediately taken up but, where doubt persists, fashion and the views of individual doctors dictate its use. Unless a clinical trial clearly demonstrates a high risk or benefit, practice is little altered. The trial of treatment for mild to moderate hypertension will almost certainly leave a large measure of uncertainty, a grey area where a decision to treat or not to treat will be a matter of opinion. It is going to be enormously expensive and I doubt whether it will alter doctors' behaviour significantly. Would it not be better to use this large sum of money for something else?

Eisenberg: What we know about the principles of learning seems to apply to the difficulty we face with physicians. If a doctor is treating a condition which is uniformly fatal, or almost so, and a new drug is introduced which is clearly beneficial, its adoption in practice is widespread and immediate—streptomycin for tuberculous meningitis is one example. But when doctors and patients are confronted with a chronic condition whose consequences are long deferred, both of them require some intermediate feedback of information sufficient to reinforce and maintain the desired behaviour. A medical audit might indeed provide just that. If, after a trial, a drug is shown to make a difference, we could look at medical practice and give doctors 'points' for behaving well. We would then be reinforcing the desired medical behaviour. We are still left with the problem of the patient, who still has to be persuaded even if the doctor does all the right things. Scientific training for medical students is certainly desirable, but to expect training given in the undergraduate curriculum to be durable in its effects is rather naive. We have to look at the organization of medical practice after the physician finishes training to see what we can build into it which will reinforce desirable behaviours and inhibit those we consider undesirable. Most of the time the doctor takes an episodic view. He has a complainant in his office, it is a busy surgery, and if he can produce temporary relief he is quite satisfied. Physicians, in their choice of a consultant, are likely to ask no further questions if the troublesome patient simply does not come back again. They often do not find out whether the specialist has helped the patient. Since placebos give symptomatic relief, and since the consequences of hypertension are long delayed (and not apt to be blamed on the physician), we need some intermediate means for reinforcing preferred behaviour. Audit may be the system, the behaviour of peers, and criticism from colleagues. In a teaching hospital medical students are wonderful instructors for physicians. One hates to be embarrassed by not being familiar with what has happened recently, or be picked up on an error. Out in general practice there is very little access to such information.

Dollery: Medical training and perhaps the whole ethos of medicine is much more oriented towards the acute emergency, the short-term situation, than it is to the very long-term one, where it may be impossible for the individual to measure the outcome of what he has done. If a doctor is treating somebody with acute pulmonary oedema it is easy to see whether that person is getting better or not, but somebody with high blood pressure can be treated for twenty years and then the doctor can retire without knowing whether what he did benefited the patient. That is the problem we are up against. Some kind of audit procedure must become general in medicine. It will be painful to bring in because people find it painful to be looked at critically. Most of us who apply for research grants have learned to endure that pain in return for the money we hope to get for our work. To train people who have never experienced it before to tolerate it will not be an easy exercise.

The MRC trial of hypertension is a local and contentious issue in the UK. Nevertheless it is important because it illustrates a general problem. The attitudes of people to this trial are really rather illuminating. It is a highly important endeavour and the results will be generally applicable. But I am interested, and at the same time rather worried, that people like Dr Bull and Dr Owen, whose opinion I very much respect, take such a strongly contrary view.

As Dr Eisenberg implied earlier, most episodes of illness are self-limiting, so whether one gives a placebo or nothing the illness will get better of itself. There are now, however, an increasing but still very small number of illnesses where people will not get better if one just gives a placebo, and where it does make some difference if one gives an effective medicine. The problem, particularly for the general practitioner, is that he still has an overwhelming noise level in relation to a relatively small signal. To get him to concentrate his mind on the signal when he is confronted with all this noise is very difficult. The trend of current practice is to emphasize situations where cure is not possible and where tender loving care is most important. There are some situations where tender loving care needs technological, scientific and intellectual support.

In therapeutics one can see this dilemma between basic research and applied research very clearly. We have neglected the applied research and it does worry me that some of the 'hard' scientists feel that the applied area is not for them. It used to be said of the MRC that it regarded phenomena made by God as being its affair and phenomena made by men as being the affair of the Ministry of Health. I don't agree with that myself!

References

[1] JOHNSON, D. A. W. (1973) Treatment of depression in general practice. *British Medical Journal 2*, 18-20
[2] SEVITT, S. & GALLAGHER, N. G. (1959) Prevention of venous thrombosis and pulmonary embolism in injured patients. *Lancet 2*, 981-989
[3] MORRIS, G. K. & MITCHELL, J. R. A. (1976) Personal communication – from paper being prepared for *Quarterly Journal of Medicine*
[4] KINCAID-SMITH, P., MCMICHAEL, J. & MURPHY, E. A. (1958) The clinical course and pathology of hypertension with papilloedema (malignant hypertension). *Quarterly Journal of Medicine 27*, 117-153
[5] DOLLERY, C. T., BULPITT, C. J., DARGIE, H. J. & LEIST, E. (1976) The care of patients with 'malignant hypertension' in London 1974-75, in *A Question of Quality*, Nuffield Provincial Hospitals Trust/Oxford University Press, London
[6] COCHRANE, A. L. (1972) *Effectiveness and Efficiency: Random Reflections on Health Services* Nuffield Provincial Hospitals Trust, London
[7] University Group Diabetes Program (1971) Effect of hypoglycaemic agents on vascular complications in patients with adult-onset diabetes. II: Clinical implications of UGDP results. *Journal of the American Medical Association 218*, 1400-1410
[8] The Coronary Drug Project (1975) Clofibrate and niacin in coronary heart disease. *Journal of the American Medical Association 231*, 360-381
[9] DOLLERY, C. T. (1971) The quality of health care, in *Challenges for Change* (McLachlan, G. ed.), pp. 5-32, Nuffield Provincial Hospitals Trust/Oxford University Press, London

Discussion: Research and the cost of treatment

Dornhorst: What is meant by the cost of treatment? Obviously it includes drugs and appliances, and the cost of any operations, admissions or outpatient attendances specifically entailed by the treatment. This may sound a straightforward calculation, but in practice it involves much guesswork in assessing the cost of the service elements.

However, if we take into account the total economic position of the patient, we are in much greater difficulties. Almost any treatment that maintains in useful employment someone who would otherwise be unable to work is likely to prove a good bargain. Thus if a person with severe haemophilia can be kept at work, £1000 spent on cryoprecipitate will have been well spent. Most people would agree that this type of calculation was proper.

But what of patients who have retired, and are net consumers rather than generators of wealth? In strict economic terms, the more effective the treatment the greater the cost to the country. Even if we ignore the increased call on pension funds and on social services, longer survival of such patients will on average lead to greater demands on the health service for conditions other than that originally treated. At this point many people begin to feel uncomfortable at the attempt to derive total costings, and perhaps the application to individual treatments is inappropriate; but as a large and increasing proportion of the hospital population is elderly, the effect on the total health service budget cannot be ignored.

I suspect that the influence of research on the total cost of treatment is not great. It is true that some expensive regimens, such as those for acute leukaemia, have been developed, but against these must be set the savings in hospital admissions achieved by many effective drugs. Antituberculous therapy and tricyclic antidepressants alone must have saved many thousands of patient-years of hospital time. The cost of some appliances is considerable, but when

89

averaged over their useful life is less alarming. Thus the current cost of a cardiac pacemaker is about £ 100 a year, which does not seem a lot to pay for what is often a return from a restricted to a full life.

The increasing scope of surgery, for example the development of coronary bypass, may create large financial demands; but these come about largely by the gradual improvement of surgical technique rather than as a result of what is usually meant by medical research.

Whatever the outcome of calculations based on such considerations, it must be viewed against a background of the widespread use of unnecessary, ineffective or needlessly expensive drugs or physical treatment, and of extravagant investigation and unnecessary hospital attendance. Research cannot be blamed for uncritical medical practice.

Black: In the UK the direct cost of research, including MRC transfer funds, voluntary foundations and so on, amounts to some 2% of the total cost of health services. Costs are easy to estimate, but in assessing benefits one runs into precisely the kind of difficulty you have just mentioned, Dr Dornhorst. A 'cure' may be produced, but it may be medicated survival rather than a real cure, and there will be further costs later so although costs are easy to assess, benefits are practically impossible. The Department of Health and Social Security certainly deplores the escalating costs.

Rogers: At the DHSS we spent a lot of time and effort trying to estimate benefits in cost terms. So far I must confess that reliable answers have totally eluded us. The attempt is worth while but at the moment one really has to use sensible judgement rather than elaborate economic calculations.

Black: It does not necessarily save money to send patients out of hospital quickly. Robert Platt once said that the cheapest way to run a hospital would be to fill it with an elderly and undemanding population, and keep people there indefinitely.

Woodruff: With expensive methods of treatment such as haemodialysis, one has to consider not only the benefit to the patients who get the kind of disease which needs that treatment, but also the assurance the rest of the population receives in knowing that if they get that sort of condition treatment will be available. Such assurance is an important component in any kind of health care service.

Beeson: I think Dr Hiatt and I would take violent issue with the idea that medical research has not skyrocketed the cost of medical care.

Hiatt: We now are beginning to realize that money spent for one kind of medical care may mean that less is available for others. This makes it particularly incumbent on us to examine not only cost–benefit aspects of a given procedure, but the comparative costs and benefits of other procedures. In the competition for resources we all agree that it is essential to be rid of procedures from which there is no benefit. An example of the latter often cited in the US is gastric freezing for peptic ulcer, which was widely used during the 1960s despite the absence of satisfactory evidence of benefit. However, it was a decade before it was finally abandoned. Surely, many other procedures now widely practised are used inappropriately and in excess.

Trials are of course useful, though expensive, but we must ask how much more expensive it will be if we don't do trials. We must also develop alternative methods for evaluation. In the US at present coronary artery bypass surgery and the computerized axial tomograph (CAT; the EMI-scanner) examinations are examples of extremely expensive procedures that are being widely used without adequate evaluation. Had Dr Dollery told us that last year forty thousand people with coronary disease were each given a pill costing over $ 10000 and causing a mortality rate of up to 12%, although neither the effectiveness nor the safety of that pill had been adequately studied, we would probably have called the police. But in the US we can make such a statement about a surgical procedure, for which we don't require four phases of a trial, or even one.

In the UK system, could payment for an unproven procedure be withheld as one way of controlling its use? If we in the medical profession don't ourselves find methods to control such procedures, we may reach a situation analogous to what may have preceded the establishment of the Food and Drug Administration in the US. Because inadequate restraints had been imposed by the profession, a bureaucracy was created then that has major advantages from the point of view of safety. However, it also has undesirable features that we can perhaps avoid if we are wiser this time.

Black: It is important to look at costs in terms not just of drugs but also of manpower, which is the most expensive resource in health services. In a way the cost of manpower is much more important, though of course they are both important.

Campbell: Dr Hiatt's last remark is extremely important. Somebody is going to have to require accountability both for fiscal reasons and for moral reasons. The coronary bypass situation is intolerable in a civilized society. If the profession does not accept the responsibility of regulating such matters, people much less well informed, using much cruder tools, are going to act instead.

Black: The established practice of the DHSS is that matters that touch on individual clinical decisions are not things for the Department to take a lead in. As a clinician I wonder how tenable this position is in the long term, and what my clinical colleagues here think of that?

Owen: This is really the central dilemma. We have a *laissez faire* system in the UK too, because of the sacred concept of clinical freedom. It is not really possible for the DHSS to dictate in any real way what doctors shall or shall not do. I wonder how long that situation can continue.

Black: We have the same problem with medical audit.

Querido: With such a general approach I do not think that one can make cost control operational. The problem is that a complicated system of enormous size is threatened by rising costs. Everybody agrees that the costs cannot be reduced and that the only thing that can be achieved is to prevent or penalize further rises. One either has to reallocate funds or forbid certain interventions or procedures. In the complicated health care system one needs to know first which subsystems offer the most sensitive points. Drugs may cost 10% of the total but human effort costs 70%. So one would like to know whether the rises are due to the increased wages of personnel, to increased numbers of personnel, to investment, or to the increased use of materials.

Dornhorst: In the UK about three-quarters of the money is spent by hospitals, largely on wages and salaries, and largely for ancillary staff, including porters and cooks. One reason for the sharply increased cost is that until recently everybody in the hospital service in the UK was underpaid. Now that has caught up with us suddenly. Against that, the number of equipped beds has come down, which means that more efficient use is made of them. Even more efficient use could still be made of them and the profession has to turn its attention to this. Some areas, such as physiotherapy, are highly labour-intensive and I think there is considerable waste here.

It is true that early discharge does not automatically save money. If extra district nurses have to be provided the cost has to be offset against any saving in hospital costs. Nevertheless, if people can go home earlier, fewer equipped beds are needed, and fewer porters, cooks and all the rest. Sir Douglas Black made the important point that this can be taken too far, as has happened to some extent in psychiatry. The effect may be that a mother or wife has to give up her work, causing absolute disruption in the family.

The EMI-scanner is certainly a major breakthrough and it saves a lot of other investigations which are not quite as expensive. Here again the capital costs are the great problem. They have to be offset against the saving in arteriography and air encephalography, which take a lot of time and are very unpleasant to the patient. Clinicians must accept that they cannot all have a scanner in their back yard. There will have to be a few regional centres and patients will have to be selected for such investigation. This is something we can do in the UK, though it may be more difficult in the US.

Hiatt: The scanning procedure is certainly important and useful. It seems likely, however, that many people are already using it much more frequently than indicated. Clearly, it is easy to order a scan for, say, a headache or a minor head injury, although in the past we would never have thought of doing an angiogram for the same condition.

I agree that one good reason for increased costs is that hospital personnel are being paid more appropriately. However, an unsatisfactory cause of increased costs is that we often use highly specialized and expensive facilities where less specialized facilities would do. For example Griner compared patients with pulmonary oedema treated in intensive care units with those who, in the previous two or three years, had been treated in regular hospital facilities.[1] Recovery rates, mortality rates, and time spent in hospital were about the same, but costs for the patients in the intensive care units were, of course, much higher. This is a problem not of technology, but of its misuse.

Dornhorst: The profession, especially the teachers, have to concentrate on this. My motto is care rather than intensity.

Pickering: This discussion shows that controlled clinical trials are cheap; for the controlled trial is just a method of arranging therapy so that its efficacy or otherwise can be displayed. When patients are sick they go to the doctor, who treats them either on the basis of knowledge, or according to what he read in the previous week's *Lancet,* or what his doctor friend said to him about a patient he saw the previous week, or the lecture he last listened to. This is what one might call random therapy, based on ignorance. It is what is being done, for example, with coronary bypass surgery at the moment. It was what was done with sympathectomy, and we never really learned how much benefit sympathectomy conferred on patients with high blood pressure. There is no doubt at all that, particularly in the US, large numbers of patients with moderate increases in arterial pressure are being given drugs to bring the pressure down. One of those drugs, reserpine, produces depression. Some, though not many, of those patients will commit suicide, and some will go into mental institutions. Some of my most grateful patients are the ones I rescued from α-methyldopa, a therapy which is often prescribed on the basis of ignorance.

Although the MRC trial to which Dr Dollery referred (p. 80) is bound to be expensive, it is not going to be nearly as expensive as the irrational distribution of drugs. The most economical piece of clinical science ever done in the UK was the trial of antituberculous drugs.[2] That beautiful piece of work established the extent to which streptomycin worked, and how far isoniazid and para-aminosalicylic acid improved its efficacy. There was no waste of life or money.

Saracci: Economists such as Feldstein[3] have indicated that, within a health insurance system, the demand for hospital services is highly sensitive to technical novelty. If new and expensive products and processes are supplied, they will be consumed. A sharp distinction should be made between novelties and the end-products of what we would call respectable research. Novelties come from invention of gadgets, from variants to existing gadgets and products, and from intermediate and provisional results of research which are quickly seized on and exploited on a commercial scale. We may regard all this mass of novelties as by-products or even waste products of an ideal and respectable research stream, but this does not make them less real and effective in absorbing an increasing amount of resources.

Perutz: I wonder how much money research has actually saved the National Health Service. For instance, how much has been saved through the closure of tuberculosis hospitals that was made possible by antituberculosis drugs?

Owen: A few years ago the Office of Health Economics calculated[4] that the annual saving being achieved by the use of tuberculostatic drugs was more than the total budget for civil science; this saving could therefore be said to be financing all five research councils, the Royal Society and the British Museum of Natural History.

Perutz: It seems that antipsychotic drugs will also save the National Health Service much money by enabling most of the mental hospitals to be closed down. Many former inpatients can now be treated at home.

Black: I wish it were true that the large mental hospitals could close as rapidly as you suggest.

Berliner: Calculations in the US show that the saving produced by the use of antipsychotic drugs is quite considerable. But people are now worried about the social cost of having these patients in the population. It is one of those things where cost and benefit are not commensurable.

Rogers: Care in the community is not necessarily cheaper than care in hospital. Also, sadly, some patients have been discharged prematurely, with tragic results. Both in terms of quality of life and in direct cost it is a difficult equation to solve.

Dollery: At a recent meeting of the Chief Scientist's research committee there was a long discussion about how research priorities could be decided. Some of the sociologists present seemed to be quite clear that they knew how to do this. Their argument seemed to be as follows, though I may have got it wrong. The cost of a complete day's suffering is called X; if the suffering is mild one can say that it is 10% of X. Y is the number of people in the community who suffer from that condition; Z is the number of days per year they are afflicted by it, and P is the probability that a particular research project will succeed in reducing that suffering. For each research proposal the sum $X \times Y \times Z \times P$ can be worked out to give a cost factor; then the proposals can be ranked by their cost. At the most superficial level this is little more than common sense, but what worries me is the uncertainty attached to most of the figures, especially the probability of success.

Beeson: It does not seem sensible to allocate research money on this kind of basis. It ought to be allocated on the basis of the probability of success, the solubility of the problem. There is no use saying we will put a lot of money into geriatric medicine or into mental health unless we have some leads. As Dr Dickinson said earlier, clinical investigation for the last twenty years has consisted mainly of measuring the failure of vital organs such as the kidney, heart or lungs. We have learned a great deal about how to make measurements of the various stages of disease, and we have also learned how to compensate for some failing functions, with the artificial kidney, respiratory support, coronary bypass surgery and so on. But now we are at the uncomfortable stage where we can prolong life but can do comparatively little in the way of curative medicine. Our priorities ought to be in the direction of really fundamental understanding and things that may lead to something better than halfway technology. People can be kept alive today who ten years ago would have died within hours, and they may then require an enormous amount of expensive therapy. I am not entering the debate about the ethical worth of prolonging life in this way, but I know that it is an important factor in the recent rapid rise in cost of medical care.

References

[1] GRINER, P. F. (1972) Treatment of acute pulmonary edema: conventional or intensive care? *Annals of Internal Medicine 77*, 501-506

[2] Medical Research Council (1948-1953) Investigations on the chemotherapy of pulmonary tuberculosis. *British Medical Journal, 2*, 769, 1948; *2*, 1073, 1950; *1*, 1157, *2*, 735, 1952; *1*, 521, 1953

[3] FELDSTEIN, M. S. (1973) The medical economy. *Scientific American 229*, 151-159

[4] Office of Health Economics, London, personal communication

Problem-solving in science

MICHAEL WOODRUFF

Department of Surgery, University of Edinburgh Medical School

Abstract Problem-solving is a characteristic activity of scientists. *Theoretical* problems are formulated as a consequence of scientists' thirst for knowledge, and their solutions take the form of general propositions, termed *hypotheses*, which are consistent with, and provide provisionally satisfactory explanations of, empirical observations. *Practical* problems appear as the result of feedback from the extra-scientific world of everyday life, industry and professional practice. Their solutions provide an improved basis for decision-making in terms of existing options or increase the number of options from which a choice may be made. The categories theoretical and practical are not mutually exclusive: practical problems often generate interesting theoretical problems, and the solution of a theoretical problem may entrain the solution of a host of practical problems.

All hypotheses are provisional because it is impossible to establish the truth of a generalization by rigorous deduction from any number of particular instances, though a single instance may suffice to refute it. This asymmetry forms the basis of Popper's analysis of scientific methodology. This analysis, though acceptable in the main, is open to criticism in the following respects: (1) it ignores the contribution to scientific progress made by unplanned perceptions; (2) it ignores the contribution of hypotheses which do not generate testable predictions; (3) it does not do justice to the extra-logical component in knowing (Polanyi's *tacit dimension*); and (4) its treatment of practical problems is inadequate.

I shall use the word *problem* to denote a question, the answer to which is not immediately obvious, which forms the starting point for, or arises in the course of, a scientific enquiry.

We may note in passing that the meaning of the word is often extended to include difficulties faced by living organisms, both individually and collectively, when neither the difficulty nor the solution is expressed in words. According to this usage the evolution of the vertebral column, or of photosynthesis, constitutes the solution of a problem; so does the action of a man who climbs

a tree to escape being eaten by a tiger—a spectacular variant, if you like, of
solvitur ambulando. Such phenomena may, of course, be of scientific interest;
in this event, however, explicit questions are formulated and explicit answers
are sought, so we come back to the point from which we started.

Problem-solving, or at any rate attempting to solve problems, is thus a
characteristic activity of scientists; indeed it may be said that all scientific
research is of this nature, though the converse is clearly not true. Let me hasten
to add that I have not overlooked the fact that the precise formulation of
problems is an important element in research, but the question of how best to
do this is itself a problem. This however is not the real starting point, for we
must first recognize that there is something to be explained, and feel that it is
worth spending time and energy in examining it more closely. I shall return
later to the question of how we do this, but would like first to look at the kinds
of problem which scientists try to solve. It is convenient to consider
these under two headings, *theoretical* problems and *practical* problems,
although, as we shall see later, these categories are by no means mutually
exclusive.

Theoretical problems are formulated as a consequence of scientific curiosity
—the thirst for knowledge, if you prefer such an expression—and their solutions
take the form of general propositions, commonly called *hypotheses*, which are
consistent with, and provide provisionally satisfactory explanations of, empirical observations, and which can often, though not always, be tested by new
experiments. I shall have occasion to refer to some examples later on. Meanwhile I would simply point out that, while writers on the philosophy of science
sometimes give the impression that the only theoretical problems worth
bothering about are those concerned with the theory of relativity or quantum
mechanics, there are plenty more to be found in other fields, both in the physical
sciences and also, of course, in biology. Indeed, since this paper forms part of
a symposium on research in medicine, most of my examples will be chosen
from medicine and biology, or from the small area of this vast field with which
I happen to be familiar.

Practical problems appear as the result of feedback from the extra-scientific
world of everyday life, industry and professional practice in engineering,
agriculture, medicine and so on. The solutions of such problems provide an
improved basis for decision-making in terms of existing options, or may actually increase the number of options from which a choice may be made. Sometimes the solution takes the form of a more or less general rule. Sometimes it
relates to a specific instance, but even then the formulation of a hypothesis is
an essential procedure because we still regularly follow the classical pattern of
syllogistic reasoning and argue from particular instance to particular instance

by way of some general proposition ('All men are mortal' is, of course, the standard example).

No one, I imagine, would deny that the solution of a theoretical problem may provide the key to the solution of a host of practical problems, though some may argue that supporting pure research is an expensive and inefficient way of contributing to the solution of practical problems. Happily, the late Vannevar Bush, in his celebrated pamphlet, *Science the Endless Frontier*,[1] has provided us with a convincing refutation of this thesis; unhappily, Bush's argument seems to have escaped the notice of some of the people responsible for the direction of scientific policy, at least in Britain.

Conversely, although it is not always appreciated by professional scientists, practical problems often generate theoretical problems of great interest and importance. Medicine provides many instances, including for example the initial development of bacteriology, virology and immunology as the result of attempts to solve the problem of prevention and treatment of infectious disease, and the recent renaissance in immunology,[2] whose origin can be traced to experiments designed to solve the clinical problem of preventing the rejection of allografts (i.e. grafts from one person to another) of skin and other tissues and organs. I have no reason to doubt that similarly striking examples could be provided by workers in other fields such as engineering and agriculture.

Let us now examine the methods by which scientists try to solve their problems, and in particular how they come to formulate and test their hypotheses.

An essential feature of all hypotheses is that they are provisional. This is a consequence of the fact that it is impossible to establish the truth of a universal generalization by rigorous deduction from any number of particular instances. or, as Einstein[3] expressed it, 'concepts have reference to sensible experiences, but they are never, in a logical sense, deducible from them'. We may note in passing that the same sort of limitation may apply even when the number of instances is infinite; it is easy to show, for example, that there is an infinity of even numbers, and not much more difficult to show that there is an infinity of primes, but it does not follow that all numbers are even or that all are prime.

There is another reason of a more subtle kind why science will always, in principle, be in need of new hypotheses. This necessity, as Polanyi[4] and Bronowski[5] have pointed out, arises from an inherent limitation of the logical sufficiency of symbolic language, which was first demonstrated in 1930 by Kurt Gödel.[6] In all such languages which are sufficiently rich to include arithmetic, it is possible, as Gödel showed, to construct sentences such that neither they nor their negations can be formally derived from the axioms of the system, if those axioms are consistent. If S is such a sentence then the sentence 'S cannot be formally derived' and also the sentence 'the consistency of the system can be formally derived' are themselves of this nature. The first sentence however is easily seen to be true, so we may add it to our system of axioms, though it cannot be deduced from those with which we started; the second sentence makes it impossible to exclude *ab initio* the possibility of hidden contradictions. Hence, as Bronowski[7] has put it, 'an axiomatic system cannot be made to generate a description of the world which matches it fully, point for point: at some points there will be holes which cannot be filled in by deduction, and at other points two opposite deductions may turn up'.

While we can never be certain of the truth of a hypothesis, we can sometimes demonstrate that it is false, because even a single instance in which it breaks down suffices logically to refute it. This asymmetry, which was first pointed out to me many years ago (certainly not later than my first year as an undergraduate) seems to me self-evident. What continues to intrigue me is why some philosophers like J. S. Mill appear to have believed that one can move from what is known empirically to what is unknown by a rigorous logical process; why so acute a thinker as Hume, though he did not make this mistake, was so deeply puzzled; and what are the implications for scientists of rejecting the myth that induction (in the philosophers' sense of the term*) is a rigorous logical process.

It is here that I have found Karl Popper[8,9,10] illuminating. I am not persuaded that he has, as he has claimed, 'solved the problem of induction', for, in so far as there is a problem and it has been solved, the solution would appear to antedate him. But he has thrown light on why there has been so much muddle-headed thinking, and has made a systematic analysis of what he has called *the logic of scientific discovery*.[9]

Popper's views on how science proceeds are summarized in the following scheme:

$$P_1 \rightarrow TT \rightarrow EE \rightarrow P_2$$

where P_1 is the initial problem, TT the first tentative theory (hypothesis), EE the process of error elimination by empirical observation, and P_2 the problem as it emerges from the first critical attempt at a solution.

It is important to notice that in this scheme the formulation of a hypothesis precedes the process of observation. Popper is insistent that 'at every instant of our pre-scientific or scientific development we are living in the centre of ... a horizon of expectations. ... This plays the part of a frame of reference: only their setting in this frame confers meaning or significance on our experiences,

---

* Mathematical induction, i.e. the process by which a proposition is shown to be true for all positive integers by showing *(a)* that *if* true for an integer *n then* it is true for *n* + 1, and *(b)* that it *is* true for some integer, is quite different, and is of course perfectly rigorous.

actions or observations ... In science it is observation rather than perception which plays the decisive part. But observation is a process in which we play an intensively active part. An observation is a perception, but one which is planned and prepared.'[8]

This analysis—whose author has been acclaimed by Sir Peter Medawar[11] as 'our foremost methodologist of science', and which, as Medawar has pointed out, accords well with the view of the role of hypotheses in scientific investigation expressed long before by Claude Bernard[12] in the introduction to his monumental work, *L'Étude de la Médecine Expérimentale*—would, I suspect, be accepted as substantially correct by most contemporary scientists. It is, however, in my view, open to criticism in two respects.

Firstly it appears to ignore the by no means negligible contribution to scientific progress made by unplanned perceptions. Fleming's[13] discovery of the effect of accidental contamination of a culture of *Staphylococci* with the mould *Penicillium notatum* seems to have been entirely unplanned, but no one would dispute its momentous consequences. Fortune, as Pasteur is said to have said, favours the prepared mind; but the preparation may have been entirely non-specific. It would be ungrateful as well as unrealistic to deny the existence of serendipity.

Secondly, Popper appears to ignore also the contribution of hypotheses which do not generate testable predictions by which they could at the time, or perhaps ever, be falsified. Michael Polanyi[14] says there have been many hypotheses of this kind which have greatly influenced scientific thought and development, including, he claims, the statistical interpretation of quantum mechanics that we owe to Max Born, and the Darwinian theory of evolution. I am tempted to add another example which is closer to my own scientific interests. As you will know, various hypotheses have been proposed to account for the great diversity of antibody-forming cells, but they all fall under one or other of two broad headings: *elective theories*, which are based on an essentially Darwinian approach to populations not of plants, animals or people, but of cells in a single organism; and *instructive theories*, which it is perhaps not unduly fanciful to regard as analogous to the Lamarckian approach to evolution. Today most immunologists would seem to opt for an elective hypothesis but, despite many attempts, no experiments have yet been designed which in my view enable us to say with confidence that one or other theory is false.

Even if Popper's approach is modified to take account of these criticisms, as it can be quite easily, we are left with the nagging question of how hypotheses come into being. There is in general no determinate method, no algorithmic procedure, 'no road, royal or otherwise' as Popper[10] says, which leads of necessity from a given set of specific facts to any universal law.

It is instructive to compare the task of the scientist with the problem of decision-making in games of various kinds. In simple games the outcome may be determined from the very beginning if both players play correctly. In noughts and crosses the result is then a draw, but if one player makes a mistake the other can make a move which is certain to lead to a win unless the second player himself makes a mistake later on. In the game of Nim a draw is impossible but it is determined from the beginning who will win if both players are sufficiently familiar with binary arithmetic to avoid making mistakes;[15] that is, depending on the initial position, *either* the first player can force a win *or* whatever move the first player makes the second will be able to force a win. The same might conceivably be true in chess if the players were capable of carrying out the necessary analysis but in practice no players, even if they have the assistance of a computer, come anywhere near to meeting this criterion, though it is beginning to be possible to do this if we consider only end-game situations. It may be remarked in passing that chess highlights the need for distinguishing between the total amount of information inherent in a particular situation, for example the disposition of the men on the board at any given stage in the game, and the information which can be retrieved in a period of time short enough for it to be turned to account. Donald Michie,[16] who so far as I know was the first to draw attention to this distinction, refers to this usable fraction of the total information as *useful knowledge*.

In science, as in ordinary life, the situation is fundamentally different, in that while we may make use of algorithmic procedures we can never in principle solve our problems by such methods alone. We depend on what in current jargon are termed *heuristic* methods; the making, as Polikarov[17] has put it, of 'plausible but fallible guesses to what is the best thing to do next'.

How do we make such guesses? How do we enunciate general laws, which not only we ourselves, but others also, find illuminating? When faced with these questions people answer with words like *inspiration, intuition,* or *instinctive reasoning*, but they sometimes do so rather shamefacedly and with the feeling that they are departing from the rigorous objectivity proper to a scientist. The very phrase *instinctive reasoning*, for example, suggests an attempt, conscious or unconscious, to confer a kind of respectability by association. And is it too far fetched to wonder whether the same explanation might apply to Popper's statement that it is *rational* to choose the best tested theory as a basis for practical action (a subject I shall return to later) when he himself insists that there can be no good reason for expecting that this or any other theory will in practice be a successful choice? Yet our only means of escape from the nightmare of solipsism is by the exercise of an extra-logical faculty, whatever we may choose to call it—and, unless we do escape, this discussion and indeed this symposium are completely illusory. Why then should we boggle at the notion that this is how we formulate hypotheses, how we choose between one hypothesis and another when neither can be shown to be false, and—to return to a question which I asked previously but did not answer—how we choose the problems we are going to try to solve?

Polanyi has referred to the extra-logical component in knowing as the *tacit dimension*[4,18,19,20] because his theory of knowledge is based on the proposition —the *fact*, he calls it—that we can know more than we can say. I am far from sure that the simple examples he cites, such as the fact that we know a person's face and can recognize it among a thousand, indeed among a million, yet usually cannot tell how we know, are of much significance today, because our capacity to analyse complex patterns and discern the essential features by which they may be recognized has advanced to the point where it is by no means inconceivable that a program could be written which would enable a computer coupled to a television camera to recognize one person out of a thousand or indeed a million. But the essence of Polanyi's thesis, or so it seems to me, is that either we know nothing or else we know a great deal more than we can prove by observation and logical deduction, and this is not invalidated by actual or foreseeable developments in pattern recognition any more than a non-mechanistic interpretation of the universe was invalidated, despite what some people may have thought at the time, by Wohler's synthesis of urea or by the cracking of the genetic code. The modern computer is no more to be feared in this context than Laplace's demon, though no doubt my colleague Donald Michie would regard the computer as of vastly greater potential intelligence. In my view, however, the great importance of Polanyi's work lies not so much in the theory of knowledge which he has propounded, for in its essentials this seems to me inescapable, as in the trenchant way in which he has defended this theory when many who find it distasteful would have preferred to ignore it; and in the illuminating comparison he has drawn between the integration of perceptions which we ordinarily take for granted but without which the external world would appear totally incoherent, and the process by which scientists 'perceive in nature the presence of lasting shapes'.[4]

The question then arises of whether a scientist's capacity to achieve this kind of knowing can be developed. I believe that it can, by education in the general sense described by Cardinal Newman in the *Idea of a University*,[21] and by unremitting devotion to the search for truth in scientific enquiry. I need scarcely add that this belief is itself, of course, not susceptible of proof by observation and deductive reasoning.

I want now to say something about the ways in which hypotheses may be tested, i.e. the *design of experiments*, and the ways in which they may have to be modified after an experiment has been performed, i.e. the *interpretation of results*. It may help to clarify the discussion, however, if we examine first some of the forms which scientific hypotheses may take, for they are not all of the same kind.

Let us begin with what is often called the *null hypothesis*, i.e. the assertion that the results observed are entirely random. I shall not attempt to define what is meant by random, but will venture the suggestion that the null hypothesis is unique in that, while it shares with other hypotheses the property of being formally unprovable, it differs from them in that it is also, in principle, not refutable. For to refute the null hypothesis would be logically equivalent to proving that the observed results were non-random. The null hypothesis is thus a sort of anti-hypothesis. Its importance lies in its widespread use as the basis of tests of statistical inference, about which I shall have something to say later.

The simplest alternative to the null hypothesis is the generalized description of what Kneale[22] calls *uniformities of nature*. Kneale refers to such descriptions as *laws*, and further subdivides them into the following convenient, though not necessarily either exhaustive or mutually exclusive, categories:

(1) Laws describing the uniform association of attributes; e.g. 'common salt is soluble in water'.

(2) Laws describing uniformity of development in certain natural processes; e.g. descriptions of embryonic development, and the second law of thermodynamics.

(3) Laws describing functional relationships between measurable quantities; e.g. the law $PV = kT$ relating the pressure (P) and volume (V) of a gas to the absolute temperature (T).

(4) Laws concerned with numerical constants in nature; e.g. the speed of light, and Avogadro's number.

When a law concerned with measurable quantities is expressed in such a way as to include a subsidiary hypothesis concerning the magnitude of the error in any of the quantities expressed, it is often referred to as a statistical hypothesis. This term is also used in a somewhat different sense to denote hypotheses which relate to the behaviour of populations of entities of various kinds, from elementary particles to people, but which say nothing about the behaviour of any particular member of the population; but the form of the hypothesis and the context should make it clear which type of statistical hypothesis is under discussion.

Hypotheses of a higher order are postulated to explain the simpler kind we have referred to as laws, and to reduce the number of independent laws by relating one law to another. Hypotheses of this kind are sometimes also called theories, but, as Medawar[23] has said, this wastes a good word. A theory is a cluster of coherent hypotheses or, in Medawar's words, 'the whole system of statements comprising hypotheses and the statements they entail'.

Let us look now at procedures we use in testing a hypothesis.

In the first place, we may, and often do, repeat an experiment under conditions which we try to make as similar as possible to those which obtained previously. Of course the conditions are never precisely the same, but most scientists would, I believe, be prepared to assert that if the conditions were the same then the result would be the same too. Some people no doubt will dismiss this version of the principle of universal causation as meaningless; others may regard it as a tautology. Personally I do not think it is either, and it has the very important consequence which again, in practice, we all seem to accept, namely, that if the second set of results is not the same as the first then the difference is due either to experimental error or to some change in the experimental conditions which it becomes our problem to identify. If, for example, the hypothesis that salt is soluble in water appeared to be falsified when tested experimentally, we might ask the following questions: Are we confident (and this may not be easy to decide) that the materials we used were in fact common salt and water? Did we reach our conclusion simply on the basis that some undissolved salt remained at the end of the experiment? If so, did we tip in too much salt or was the water too cold? Only after we had exhausted obvious questions of this kind might we think of looking for more esoteric explanations. Again, if on some occasion we obtained a value for the velocity of light which differed widely from the accepted value, we would look first to see whether our apparatus was insufficiently sensitive or whether we had made a mistake in our calculations, and would be astonished if the discrepancy could not be explained in this way.

The other type of test applied to a hypothesis is one designed to test its wider implications. Experiments of this kind often test two or more hypotheses simultaneously. This makes interpretation difficult when the results observed differ from those predicted; on the other hand, in so far as it is legitimate to speak of results supporting a hypothesis, an observed result in conformity with that predicted lends support to both hypotheses. All this is no doubt obvious to anyone engaged in experimental work, but for those who are not I venture to give a simple example. It was observed by many investigators from about 1915 onwards that the capacity of animals which had been exposed to whole body X-irradiation to make antibodies to antigens of various kinds was in general less than that of animals of the same species, sex and age group that had not been irradiated, and it was therefore postulated that X-irradiation in some way interferes with the mechanism on which immunological responses depend. An experiment which further tests this hypothesis, and also the hypothesis of Medawar that allograft rejection results from an immunological reaction by the host in response to antigens in the graft, was designed and first performed in 1950 by Dempster and his colleagues, and it was found as predicted that irradiated rabbits rejected skin allografts more slowly than normal rabbits.[24]

In designing experiments one must of course consider their feasibility. Some experiments one would like to perform may not be possible, at any rate at the time, either because it has not been possible to construct the apparatus required or, as has often happened in biology, because the experimenter had not developed, or found anyone else who possessed, the necessary manipulative skill. By way of illustration we may cite, for example, the dependence of high energy physics on the development of the cyclotron and other equipment of a similar kind, the dependence of modern knowledge of cell structure on the development of the electron microscope, the dependence of many advances in immunobiology on the development of highly inbred strains of mice, and of many other advances in biology and medicine on the availability of radioactive isotopes of various kinds and appropriate counting equipment, and the dependence of advances in our understanding of the functions of lymphocytes on the development of techniques for cannulating the thoracic duct and peripheral lymphatics; but many other examples could be given. At other times repetition of an old experiment may not seem worth while because the resolving power of the methods available is little or no greater than that of the methods used previously. Critical reappraisal of Michelson and Morley's experiment of 1887,[25] and the repetition of that experiment by D. C. Miller[26] and his colleagues over some twenty years, both of which yielded results which were not entirely compatible with the assumptions underlying the special theory of relativity,[27] had to await the availability of optical masers and lasers.[28]

If new experimental results are incompatible with a hypothesis then the hypothesis is, strictly speaking, falsified. As Jeffreys[29] has pointed out, however, since allowance must be made for errors of observation, any criterion for rejection must be quantitative. Moreover—and this is sometimes overlooked by those who discuss the methodology of science from a philosophical standpoint—the estimate of error is itself a hypothesis, and it may happen that this, rather than the hypothesis we are trying to test, is the one which is false. The curious fact, mentioned above, that at least until quite recently, measurements of the velocity of light had yielded results apparently incompatible with the special theory of relativity, and yet somehow no one seriously questioned the validity of the theory on this account, suggests that the possibility of experimental error considerably in excess of the estimated upper limit must have been widely accepted, if not explicitly then subconsciously.[4]

The situation is different with mathematical generalizations of a kind which abound in the theory of numbers[15] (for example, Fermat's 'last theorem'), which have been found to be true in a large number of instances but never proved rigorously to be generally true. Here a single instance in which the generalization failed would suffice to disprove it since the possibility of experimental error does not exist. For this reason it seems preferable to speak of such generalizations as *conjectures* and not as hypotheses.

Even when a hypothesis is falsified this of course does not imply that it is false in every particular. No logical rules can suffice to decide the extent to which it should be modified. Sometimes the discrepancy may be removed by making quite a small *ad hoc* change in the original statement which does not generate new testable predictions, and this seems to me a perfectly proper sort of modification despite the objections raised by some theorists. Of course if every change were of this kind progress would come to a standstill, but in real life there is no danger of this, for if the originator of a hypothesis is unwilling to put forward what Popper calls *bold* modifications, then sooner or later others will do so if the hypothesis relates to questions which they regard as important.

If on repeated testing over a wide range of applications a hypothesis is not falsified, our feeling of confidence in it grows. Must this always be a purely subjective judgement, or can one find objective ways of ranking alternative hypotheses, or even of assigning to each one a numerical value which is a measure of the support it has gained or the degree of confidence it merits?

It is, I think, manifestly impossible to develop a calculus of this kind which is logically rigorous and entirely reliable, but it does not follow that nothing whatever, or nothing of value, can be done. Let us therefore by all means abandon the fruitless search for a complete system of inductive inference, but let us look instead at the possibility of developing systems which have what Meltzer[30] has called the property of relative completeness, i.e. whose completeness is limited only by the data available and by the deductive power of the system used to show that the observed results are deducible from the hypothesis.

The most familiar approach to the problem is to calculate, on the basis of the null hypothesis, the mathematical probability of the whole set of observed results arising by random sampling from a hypothetical infinite population, some of whose properties (e.g. normal distribution) may be assumed *a priori*, and others of which are estimated from the observations. One can often go a step further and assign so-called *confidence limits* to estimated parameters of the population, so that one may for example speak of an estimated mean value with 95% or 99% or 99.9% confidence limits of such and such, meaning that, given the assumed population, the chance that the mean of a random sample will lie within the limits indicated are 95%, 99% and 99.9% respectively.

All this, *given the assumptions about the population*, is logically rigorous. On the other hand one cannot, from a given or assumed sample, calculate the probability that the population from which it was drawn had such and such characteristics. Therefore, unless we abandon the attempt to quantitate the support gained by a hypothesis, we shall need a new term, and the term likelihood, which derives from R. A. Fisher,[31] seems the most appropriate.

Can one define this term in such a way that one can meaningfully and usefully speak of the likelihood that a particular population was the one from which a given sample was drawn; or alternatively can one speak of the relative likelihood of various alternative hypotheses which relate to the same set of data? Edwards,[32] starting where Fisher left off, has attacked this question and has defined the likelihood, $L(H/S)$, of the hypothesis H given data S as $k\,P(S/H)$, where $P(S/H)$ is the probability of the data (regarded as a sample) arising by random sampling when H is given, and k is an arbitrary constant which is however the same for all hypotheses relating to the same data. Unlike probability, therefore, likelihood does not have an absolute value, but one can speak of the relative likelihood of various alternative hypotheses and rank them accordingly. There does not seem to be any logical objection to this definition, though whether it is consistent with the meaning of the word likelihood in ordinary conversations is of course another matter. I am inclined to think that it is, and that the calculus of likelihood, foreseen by Fisher and developed by Edwards, provides a basis for scientific inference which is as powerful as traditional tests of significance based on the null hypothesis, and less open to logical objection. Another function, $C(h,e)$, to be read as the degree of confirmation of hypothesis h by observation e, has been introduced by Popper,[9] who regards it as a generalization of Fisher's likelihood function. I doubt whether it will prove as useful a tool as Edwards' relative likelihood, partly because of its greater complexity and partly because of Popper's insistence that it can be interpreted as the degree of confirmation of h by e only if 'e reports the result of our sincere efforts to overthrow h', a requirement which, he admits, cannot be formalized.

How in the light of this discussion should we choose between competing hypotheses?

As a basis for new experiments Popper recommends choosing what he calls the *best testable* hypothesis; i.e. the one with the greatest information content and the greatest explanatory power. This sounds like excellent advice, but in practice other factors often help to determine the choice. A scientist working in a particular field, for example, often has a hunch that one among various possible hypotheses is true, and may then seek first to show that the others are false. I would add, for what such a value judgement is worth, that I personally see no objection to this, provided of course that the scientist is prepared to accept whatever new evidence he finds, irrespective of where it may lead.

In the extra-scientific world the choice is constrained in another way for, if I may paraphrase the words of Wilfred Trotter,[33] an attitude of eternal procrastination, which is a necessity for the pure scientist, is here an unaffordable luxury. The practical man, if he has any scientific insight, knows full well that there is no way by which he can be certain of making correct decisions, but he wants nevertheless a guide which, if consistently followed, will enable him to make decisions which turn out later to have been correct more often than would otherwise have been the case. Popper advises that practical decisions should be based on the *best tested* theory, and goes on to say that this is a *rational* thing to do. In this context, however, as I have already mentioned, he is not using the word rational in the familiar sense of logically deducible; what he seems to be saying is that this is the kind of choice which would earn the approval of rational people—of philosophers, if you like. While this may be good advice the reason given has little appeal for practical people. They are largely indifferent to the approval of philosophers; in the language of games they are playing to win, and, while they know that they cannot win always, they want to do so as often as possible. In so far as methods of assessing hypotheses by their relative likelihood, by Popper's function of corroboration, or by whatever other criteria may be devised, provide a guide which meets this criterion, they will appeal to practical people; if they fail to do this they will not.

In practice, whatever we may say, we base our choice, as Hume saw clearly,[34] on what we *believe* to be true. It is clearly important to adopt a highly critical attitude and to eliminate beliefs which can be shown to be false, since these are liable to trap us into making wrong decisions. On the other hand, if we try to scrap the lot and become completely agnostic we shall find ourselves totally paralysed, except perhaps, as Hume[34] found, in respect of such pleasant, but extracurricular, activities as dining, gaming, merry-making and so on. There are of course different levels of belief; what I have been referring to is belief which is so compelling that it determines our actions in matters which we regard as important. It is this which, if I understand them rightly, theologians call *faith*. Perhaps the time has come when scientists might usefully add this term to their vocabulary.

'The simple believeth every word', said the writer of the Book of Proverbs.[35] The sceptic, we might add, believes nothing. The successful problem-solver, however, is neither over-credulous nor over-sceptical. Like the proverbial prudent man he 'looketh well to his going', his actions are guided by his convictions, and he is well aware that the solution of scientific problems is not only a science but an art.

ACKNOWLEDGEMENTS

I am deeply grateful to Professors Bernard Meltzer, Donald Michie and Tom Torrance for helpful comments on the first draft of this paper. They must however be absolved from any responsibility for the opinions I have expressed.

Discussion

Black: About ten years ago someone offered the University of Manchester money for a chair of decision-making. A wise vice-chancellor persuaded him to change this to decision theory, and then of course in the end it was back to the theory of games.

The way to enable a computer to 'recognize' people may be through the art of the caricaturist, who with comparatively few lines can make a recognizable image. That kind of approach may take us further in the ability to computerize electrocardiographic tracings and so on, by picking out the essential features.

Eisenberg: I think you underestimate the problem of pattern recognition by computers. An oval can be distinguished from a circle with much greater reliability by human observers than by the best available computer program. An anthropologist in one of the Polynesian islands once asked the natives to classify the species of birds which were available on that island, using their own terminology. He then brought from a neighbouring island several intermediate forms which were not present on the first island and had never been seen there before. The people fitted these birds into their scheme on Linnaean kinds of principles. Biologists, especially classifiers and systematists, find identities which defy coherent definitions. They abstract from a series of diverse features those things which are held in common. Physicians often know what they cannot specify, and I suppose that is why we choose our physicians very carefully.

Dickinson: That seems extremely mystical. Are you suggesting that in due course computers will not distinguish circles from ovals more efficiently than unaided humans, or that the process of recognizing species of birds has a sort of intuitive component that cannot ultimately be rationalized?

Eisenberg: I have sufficient faith in science to share your belief that ultimately what is now knowable but unspecifiable will come more and more in the direction of specifiability. In the meantime I think we ignore at our peril our ability to know many more things than can be demonstrated in a rigorous sense.

Woodruff: I agree.

Dickinson: I think it was A. J. Ayer who pointed out that the most essential attribute of a scientific hypothesis is that new observations or experiments can make it more or less likely to be correct. Clearly there is some asymmetry, and one refutation carries more weight than one confirmation—but the refutation may itself be incorrect. For example, the conclusion that all swans are white is not refuted by finding one black one if the black one has been painted black.

Saracci: One should be careful not to mix up the various elements (logical, psychological, social) involved in the process of scientific discovery. This schematically goes from initial observations acting as stimuli on imagination, to hypothesis formulation, to hypothesis testing, to collective consensus on a non-rejected hypothesis. Popper[9] essentially focuses on the 'logical skeleton of the procedure of testing... hypotheses', leaving aside 'such processes' (which) 'are the concern of empirical psychology but hardly of logic'. He maps the common logical ground for inter-subjectively valid knowledge. However, beyond this logical aspect of hypothesis testing and validation the whole process needs to be looked at in terms of the psychological and, above all, social elements and forces governing its development in the real world, as the well-known working scheme put forward by T. S. Kuhn[36] does. On the other hand, inside the logical sphere itself one finds more types of scientific and testable hypotheses than just statistical hypotheses to which the 'likelihood principle' mentioned by Professor Woodruff is relevant. Indeed, as Popper himself stated with reference to his approach to providing a basis for the corroboration of hypotheses 'we can interpret ... our measure of degree of corroboration as a generalization of Fisher's likelihood function', namely a generalization outside the restricted, though in practice very important, class of statistical hypotheses.

Black: The biggest hidden assumption in the process of scientific discovery is probably that there *is* such a thing as causality and that it is universal. This is a very untestable hidden assumption.

Dickinson: Popper surely would not reject the evolutionary hypothesis as not scientific. All that one demands of a hypothesis is that it can be made more likely or less likely when evidence is assembled. That is certainly true of the evolutionary hypothesis. Popper simply rejects the idea that one can *prove* anything.

Woodruff: There must be hypotheses which at the time, at least, are not testable. But playing about with ideas can generate other ideas and I think he overlooks that.

Campbell: I think that what Popper asks is not that the hypothesis shall be falsifiable at the time it is put forward but that it should be potentially falsifiable. I would regard the theory of evolution as being potentially falsifiable.

Hjort: One practical consequence arising from Popper's thought, or Mao Tse-Tung's, is that it would make us more able to tolerate criticism. The medical profession has a very low ability to tolerate criticism, especially from people outside the profession.

Woodruff: Where there are two competing hypotheses, both refutable but only one of which is refuted, this is clearly the one we reject unless we are completely insensitive to criticism. I am not advocating that sort of insensitivity, of course. But where there are two or three possibilities, none of which at the time is refutable, then we have to choose a working hypothesis for further theoretical work, and choose a guide for practical action. We all make these choices even though they are not logically defensible, because on the information available none of the possibilities are capable of being rejected. Popper rightly draws attention to the need to look critically at things to see whether they stand up to verification. I accept that entirely, but where there are two or more possibilities that cannot be distinguished in that way, one is living in an ivory tower if one doesn't try to make a choice in some other way.

Eisenberg: Another way in which the utility of theories or hypotheses can be valued, other than by their ability to be refuted, is by whether they generate experiments, leading one to make observations or to look at phenomena in new ways. Neurology provides a rather spectacular example. F. J. Gall developed phrenology on the basis of the extant psychology which held that there were some thirty mental faculties. He assumed that the brain was like muscle and that the more it was exercised, the more hypertrophic it would become. He knew that the brain had something to do with pushing out the skull. Thus, he felt for the bumps on the skull which might reflect underlying areas of cortical hypertrophy. Then he searched for individuals who had faculties that were especially well developed. He had one colleague who was extremely proptotic (with protruding eyes) and very verbal, so he located verbal facility in the frontal lobes. He knew of a Don Juan the back of whose head was rather large and thus he located amativeness in the cerebellum. Those two particular choices proved to be rather remarkable, because the original discovery by Broca of the speech area was guided by phrenology. Broca had a patient who had a stroke and lost his power of speech. At autopsy there was a softening in the frontal lobe to which the aphasia was attributed. In fact, reexamination of that brain indicates multiple areas of softening; the choice of the proper area, later verified, was guided by phrenology. Pierre Flourens, a Belgian physiologist who disagreed with phrenology on theological grounds, lopped off the cerebella of pigeons and found that they lost their locomotive ability and their balance. (I suspect that they were not very good at courtship either.)

Falsifiability as a criterion is related to the fact that it leads to observations or data or experiments which carry one further. Medicine has numerous examples of the right discovery being made for the wrong theoretical reason, which then leads to further hypotheses. It is in the nature of human consciousness that to respond to the world in an organized fashion we need hypotheses about that world, and certainly some of them are tacit.

Phillips: Popper doesn't propose that all scientists work by first producing falsifiable hypotheses but rather that science advances in this particular way and therefore that when scientists are formulating hypotheses they should be falsifiable hypotheses.

Woodruff: Nobody would quarrel with that. My criticism of Popper is that he leaves some important things unsaid. I am not quarrelling with anything specific that he has said. There are situations when we are not in a position to reject something as falsifiable at the time, yet where we are compelled to make a choice. It is important to try and analyse the basis of the kind of choice we can make in those situations.

Phillips: But doesn't the scientific community then struggle to get propositions into a falsifiable state? Similarly, people struggle to put taxonomy into a proper numerical state but they have not yet succeeded.

Woodruff: Yes, but sometimes a conviction that a theory is correct is very profound. The scientific community can then be extraordinarily blind to observations which *prima facie* appear to falsify the theory.

References

[1] Bush, V. (1945) *Science the Endless Frontier*, Government Printing Office, Washington
[2] Woodruff, M. F. A. (1976) Renaissance of immunology, *New Zealand Medical Journal* 83, 1-4
[3] Einstein, A. (1935) *The World as I See It*, Lane, London
[4] Polanyi, M. (1958) *Personal Knowledge*, Routledge & Kegan Paul, London
[5] Bronowski, J. (1951) *The Common Sense of Science*, Heinemann, London
[6] Gödel, K. (1930) Die Vollständigkeit der Axiome des logischen Funktionenkalküls. *Monatshefte für Mathematik und Physik 37*, 349-360
[7] Bronowski, J. (1966) The logic of the mind. *Nature (London) 209*, 1171-1173
[8] Popper, K. R. (1972) *Objective Knowledge*, Clarendon Press, Oxford
[9] Popper, K. R. (1968) *The Logic of Scientific Discovery*, revised edition, Hutchinson, London (first published in 1935 as *Logik der Forschung*)
[10] Popper, K. R. (1963) *Conjectures and Refutations*, Routledge & Kegan Paul, London
[11] Medawar, P. B. (1967) *The Art of the Soluble*, Methuen, London
[12] Bernard, C. (1865) *Introduction a l'Étude de la Médecine Expérimentale*, Baillière, Paris
[13] Fleming, A. (1929) On the antibacterial action of cultures of a penicillium, with special reference to their use in the isolation of *B. influenzae*. *British Journal of Experimental Pathology 10*, 226-236
[14] Polanyi, M. (1972) Genius in science, in *Archives de L'Institut International des Sciences Théoriques*, No. 18, pp. 11-25, Office International de Librairie, Bruxelles
[15] Hardy, G. H. & Wright, E. M. (1954) *An Introduction to the Theory of Numbers*, 3rd edn., Oxford University Press, London
[16] Michie, D. (1976) A mathematical theory of advice, in *Machine Representations of Knowledge* (Elcock, W. E. & Michie, D., eds.), Reidel, Dordrecht

[17] POLIKAROV, A. (1974) Methodical and historical essays in the natural and social sciences. *Boston Studies in the Philosophy of Science 14*, 211-233
[18] POLANYI, M. (1967) *The Tacit Dimension*, Routledge & Kegan Paul, London
[19] POLANYI, M. (1969) *Knowing and Being*, Routledge & Kegan Paul, London
[20] TORRANCE, T. F. *Integration and Interpretation in Natural and Theological Science* (in preparation)
[21] NEWMAN, J. H. (1947) *Idea of a University* (Harrold, C. F., ed.), Longmans, Green & Co, London (first published in 1852, revised and expanded in 1859 and 1873)
[22] KNEALE, W. (1949) *Probability and Induction*, Oxford University Press, London
[23] MEDAWAR, P. B. (1957) *The Uniqueness of the Individual*, Constable, Edinburgh
[24] DEMPSTER, W. J., LENNOX, B. & BOAG, J. W. (1960) Prolongation of survival of skin homotransplants in the rabbit by irradiation of the host. *British Journal of Experimental Pathology 31*, 670-679
[25] MICHELSON, A. A. & MORLEY, E. W. (1887) On the relative motion of the earth and the luminiferous ether. *American Journal of Science 34*, 333-345
[26] MILLER, D. C. (1933) The ether drift experiment and the determination of the absolute motion of the earth. *Reviews of Modern Physics 5*, 203-242
[27] SHANKLAND, R. S., McCUSKEY, S. W., LEONE, F. C. & KUERTI, G. (1955) New analysis of the interferometer observations of Dayton C. Miller. *Reviews of Modern Physics 27*, 167-178
[28] JASEJA, T. S., JAVAN, A., MURRAY, J. & TOWNES, C. H. (1964) Test of special relativity of the isotropy of space by use of infra red masers. *Physical Review Series A (US) 133*, 1221-1225
[29] JEFFREYS, H. (1973) *Scientific Inference*, 3rd edn., Cambridge University Press, London
[30] MELTZER, B. (1970) The semantics of induction and the possibility of complete systems of inductive inference. *Artificial Intelligence 1*, 189-192
[31] FISHER, R. A. (1958) *Statistical Methods for Research Workers*, 13th edn., Oliver & Boyd, Edinburgh
[32] EDWARDS, A. W. F. (1972) *Likelihood*, Cambridge University Press, London
[33] TROTTER, W. (1935) General ideas in medicine. *British Medical Journal 2*, 609-614
[34] HUME, D. (1739) A treatise concerning human nature, in *British Empirical Philosophers* (1952: Ayer, A. J. and Winch, R., eds.), Routledge & Kegan Paul, London
[35] Proverbs, *XIV*, 15
[36] KUHN, T. S. (1962) *The Structure of Scientific Revolutions*, University of Chicago Press, Chicago

Fundamental research in molecular biology: its relevance to medicine

M. F. PERUTZ

MRC Laboratory of Molecular Biology, University Postgraduate Medical School, Cambridge

Abstract Any research which has shed light on the nature of disease or opened new ways to its prevention or cure is here termed relevant, and the question will be asked whether the research could have been planned with these aims in mind. Examples will be taken from the chemistry and X-ray analysis of proteins and from molecular genetics. Blow and Hartley determined the amino acid sequence and atomic structure of the digestive enzyme chymotrypsin in order to solve the problem of enzymic catalysis. They succeeded but what they found has proved to be of much wider importance than could have been foreseen at the outset: it gives the key to the mechanism of blood clotting and suggests new methods for its control. X-ray analysis of haemoglobin was started at a time when the structure of proteins was regarded as the central problem of biology, but it did not seem likely then that the results would shed light on the molecular pathology of inherited diseases. Ames made a life-long study of the genetic control of histidine biosynthesis in *Salmonella* because it represents an example of a widely used biological mechanism, but without expecting it to have any practical applications. Yet his recent exploitation of the system for the rapid and sensitive detection of chemical carcinogens may represent a breakthrough in cancer prevention. This unpredictable relationship of molecular biology to medicine is symptomatic of the subject's youth.

The activities of living cells depend mainly on two kinds of very large molecules: proteins and nucleic acids. The proteins act as biological catalysts—the enzymes; their structure is determined by nucleic acids—the genes; and their synthesis depends on an interplay of molecules of both kinds. Molecular biologists have tried to find out what proteins and nucleic acids are made of and what they look like, and this has often told them how they work. Their field touches many subjects, but borders mainly on biochemistry and genetics. The leaders in the field have often been physicists and chemists rather than biologists, but their methods have covered a wide range from mathematics to bacteriology.

115

Molecular biology is sometimes said to be of little medical significance because it has not cured anyone yet. A hundred years ago the same might have
been said of histology. At that time cellular anatomy and pathology began to
improve our understanding of many diseases; today molecular anatomy and
pathology give us much deeper insights. I shall illustrate this theme by examples
taken from four different fields of research. The first two are from the fields
with which I am most familiar, the structure and function of proteins; the second
two are from molecular genetics. I shall first show how research on the structure
of protein-digesting enzymes has led to an understanding of blood clotting and
other important functions whose relation to digestion no one had suspected.
I shall then relate how my own work on the structure of haemoglobin has
improved our understanding of genetic diseases and how basic research on
autoxidation of haemoglobin has suggested a way of treating certain inherited
anaemias. My next two themes are concerned with the effects of ultraviolet
light and chemical carcinogens on nucleic acids and their relation to human
cancer.

PROTEOLYTIC ENZYMES AND THEIR INHIBITORS

In the 1950s the structure and catalytic mechanism of enzymes still ranked
as one of the great unsolved problems in biochemistry. At that time two of my
colleagues, B. S. Hartley and D. M. Blow, became interested in the digestive
enzyme chymotrypsin, simply because they regarded it as the most hopeful and
interesting one to attack. This enzyme is made in the pancreas and is closely
related to two other pancreatic enzymes, trypsin and elastase. All three enzymes
split protein chains. Chymotrypsin splits fastest those peptide bonds that
follow amino acids with aromatic side chains, while trypsin goes for peptide
bonds that follow basic side chains, and elastase for those with very short side
chains. All three enzymes are secreted into the jejunum in the form of inactive
precursors, known as chymotrypsinogen, trypsinogen and proelastase; all three
precursors are activated by trypsin. Now the problem for the organism is that
free trypsin is an undesirable enzyme to have about outside the digestive tract
since it activates its own precursor and the precursors of other proteolytic
enzymes. Perhaps for this reason the pancreas also makes a small protein which
scavenges and inhibits any traces of free activated trypsin. This is the pancreatic
trypsin inhibitor.

Hartley[1] and his colleagues determined the amino acid sequence of chymotrypsin and chymotrypsinogen while Blow and others[2] solved the three-
dimensional structure of chymotrypsin by X-ray analysis. Other workers followed with the structure of chymotrypsinogen, of trypsin, of elastase, of the trypsin

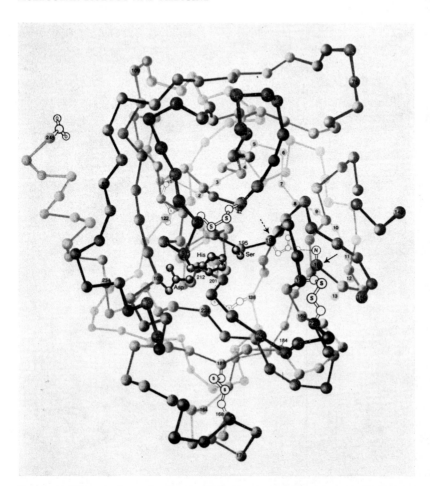

FIG. 1. Folding of the polypeptide chains in chymotrypsin. The balls represent the α-carbon atoms. The complex of aspartate, histidine and serine which constitutes the catalytic site is at the centre. The specificity pocket lies down to the right of that site. Trypsin activates the precursor, chymotrypsinogen, by cutting out residues 15 and 14. The free amino group of isoleucine 16, marked by the unbroken arrow, then forms an internal salt bridge with aspartate 194, marked by the broken arrow; this leads to the structural rearrangement which opens the specificity pocket (see Fig. 3). (Reproduced, with permission, from Stroud[3]).

inhibitor and of the trypsin–trypsin inhibitor complex. Together, Blow, Hartley and their colleagues worked out the mechanism of activation and catalysis, and Huber and Blow that of inhibition.[3]

Chymotrypsin consists of 242 amino acid residues in three separate chains, which are linked by disulphide bonds (Fig. 1). Its active site contains a serine, a histidine and an aspartate juxtaposed so that protons can shuttle backwards

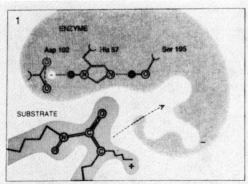

1 ENZYME

Asp 102   His 57   Ser 195

SUBSTRATE

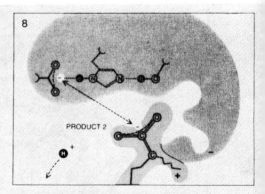

8 PRODUCT 2

H +

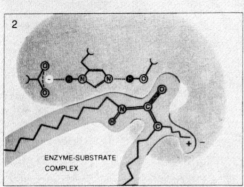

2

ENZYME-SUBSTRATE
COMPLEX

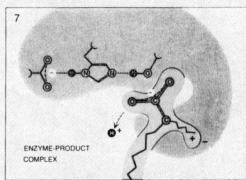

7

ENZYME-PRODUCT
COMPLEX

H +

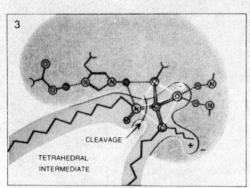

3

CLEAVAGE

TETRAHEDRAL
INTERMEDIATE

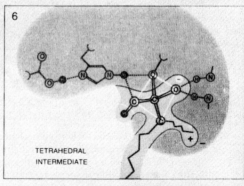

6

TETRAHEDRAL
INTERMEDIATE

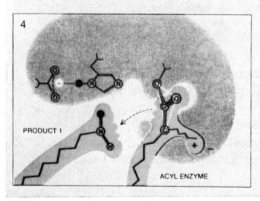

4

PRODUCT 1

ACYL ENZYME

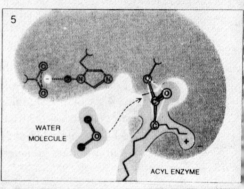

5

WATER
MOLECULE

ACYL ENZYME

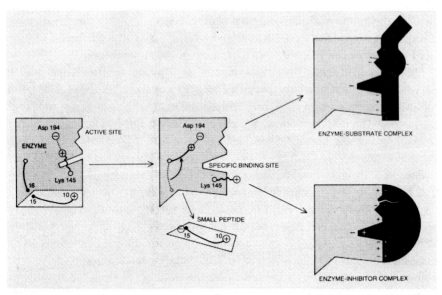

FIG. 3. *Left*: The precursor trypsinogen with closed specificity pocket. *Middle*: Trypsin activates the precursor by cutting out residues 10–15; this opens the specificity pocket. *Right top*: Complementarity of enzyme–substrate complex: the substrate is split at the broken line towards the right. *Right bottom*: Complementarity of enzyme inhibitor complex; inhibitor cannot be split and remains attached to the enzyme. (Reproduced, with permission, from Stroud.[3])

and forwards between them, forming what Hartley and Blow called a charge relay system (Fig. 2). This serves to polarize the serine side chain so that it can attack its substrate at the carbonyl carbon of the peptide bond to be split. At first a short-lived intermediate is formed in which that carbon is bonded to the seryl oxygen without a split in the peptide bond; next the peptide bond is split, and the side of the substrate carrying the free amino group is released while the other side remains attached to the enzyme with its carbonyl carbon. Finally, a hydroxyl from the ambient water replaces the serine hydroxyl at the carbonyl carbon and the remaining substrate is released by the enzyme. Now that this mechanism has been discovered, it has been found to be common to many enzymes with very different specificities and functions.

In the chymotrypsin family of enzymes the substrate is recognized by a pocket that lies next to the active site and is so tailored that it attracts the side

---

←
FIG. 2. Catalytic mechanism of trypsin. 1. The complex of aspartate 102, histidine 57 and serine 195 which constitutes the catalytic site. Down and to the right is the specificity pocket with the negative charge of aspartate 189 to attract the positively charged lysine side chain of the substrate. The other pictures are self-explanatory. (Reproduced, with permission, from Stroud[3]).

chain of the amino acid preceding the peptide bond to be split. In the inactive precursor that specificity pocket is closed. Trypsin activates the precursors by splitting their chains in a way that allows the pocket to open (Fig. 3).

The pancreatic trypsin inhibitor mimics a substrate by presenting to the enzyme a side chain which its specificity pocket recognizes, but the peptide bond following that side chain is so shielded from water that the enzyme cannot split it. Instead, the inhibitor remains firmly attached to the enzyme in a position resembling the one fleetingly occupied by a substrate at the first intermediate stage of catalysis (Fig. 3).[4,5]

The mechanisms of activation, recognition and catalysis of chymotrypsin first became known in outline in 1969, and the way in which the pancreatic trypsin inhibitor blocks trypsin in 1972; some further important details have been added since. Whenever nature has invented an effective and versatile device, it tends to exploit it over and over again for different functions. The same mechanisms of activation, recognition, catalysis and inhibition have now been found in at least four other functions: the clotting of blood, the dissolution of blood clots, the disposal of complexes of antigen and antibody by complement, and the lowering of blood pressure by the release of kinins. The raising of blood pressure by the release of angiotensins is also due to a proteolytic enzyme known as renin, but this is of a type different from trypsin, and its structure is still unknown. The interplay of protein-digesting enzymes and their inhibitors appears to be important also in degenerative diseases such as pulmonary emphysema and rheumatoid arthritis.

Suitable stimuli cause blood to clot with explosive velocity, but it hardly occurs to anyone that this process might be an example of protein digestion. It has recently been discovered that this instant response is brought about by a cascade of proteolytic enzymes.[6] Injury to a blood vessel, say, activates a few molecules of the first enzyme. Each of these molecules then activates, say, fifty molecules of the second enzyme, and so on, in a series of five steps, until an avalanche of activated thrombin converges upon the soluble fibrinogen and turns it into the insoluble fibrin (Fig. 4). It is now certain that part of the thrombin molecule has a structure which is almost identical to that of trypsin; in the clotting factors XIa, IXa and Xa the parts of the sequences that have so far been analysed are also like those of trypsin. The precursor of each of these enzymes is activated by the preceding enzyme in the clotting cascade by the same kind of mechanism by which trypsin opens the specificity pocket in trypsinogen or chymotrypsinogen, and each possesses the same charge relay system for the hydrolysis of peptide bonds. The functioning of the cascade depends on the presence of calcium ions and on nutrition with adequate amounts of vitamin K.

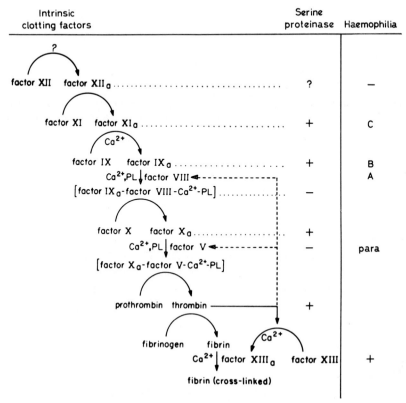

FIG. 4. Cascade of intrinsic clotting factors. Those marked + are enzymes similar to trypsin. (Reproduced, with permission, from Davie & Kirby.[6])

The clotting factors possess several refinements which the pancreatic enzymes lack. Their specificities are probably greater and they are activated not in free solution, where they would be too widely dispersed, but on the surface of phospholipid membranes of blood platelets where they are crowded together. Prothrombin, the precursor of thrombin, has an extra 274 amino acids which are not found in trypsinogen, and these form an attachment which binds it to the membrane, but only in the presence of calcium ions. On activation by factor Xa this attachment is split off and thrombin is released into the plasma. A great advance has recently been made in our understanding of the role of calcium and its dependence on vitamin K. It has been found that calcium ions are bound to prothrombin by ten residues of a new amino acid, never encountered before, γ-carboxyglutamate; the residues lie near the amino terminus of the chain. The new amino acid is made after the polypeptide chain of prothrombin has been assembled in the liver, by an enzyme system that adds a second carboxyl group to each of the first ten glutamates; and this subsidiary enzyme system that adds carboxyl groups requires vitamin K as a cofactor. In the clotting cascade, the other three trypsin-like factors or enzymes also require calcium in order to be activated, which implies that they are subject to the same vitamin K-dependent modification as prothrombin. These discoveries explain how vitamin K antagonists interfere with blood clotting: by reducing the calcium affinity of prothrombin and of three other clotting factors the antagonists prevent these factors from binding to the phospholipid membrane and thereby inhibit their activation.[7]

The therapeutic uses of vitamin K antagonists were discovered long before its mode of action was understood, but the new discoveries will allow the antagonists to be applied more rationally and with greater knowledge of their possible side effects. For example, the presence of the new amino acid γ-carboxyglutamate in prothrombin suggested that it might be worth searching for it in other calcium-binding proteins. This search has led to the amino acid being isolated from a protein in the bones of the 14-week-old chick, which suggests that γ-carboxyglutamate may be needed for the deposition of calcium in developing bones;[8] this explains why treatment of women during the first three months of pregnancy with anticoagulants of the dicoumarol type has led to bone anomalies in the fetus.

There are at least two natural anticoagulants which keep clotting under control. An excess of free thrombin in the plasma stops activation of more prothrombin by splitting off its first 156 residues, thus detaching it from the phospholipid membrane before it can be activated. A plasma inhibitor, AIII antithrombin, inhibits thrombin and other clotting factors by a mechanism apparently similar to that by which the pancreatic inhibitor blocks trypsin, except that by itself AIII antithrombin acts much more slowly. It has recently been found that heparin exerts its instant anticlotting effect by accelerating the reaction of AIII antithrombin with thrombin and with the other factors. Patients with a congenital deficiency of AIII antithrombin have an increased tendency to thrombosis,[9] which shows that this inhibitor is an essential part of the checks and balances in the clotting system.

AIII antithrombin is one of six different antiproteinases so far discovered in human plasma. Another of the six that has recently assumed medical importance is α_1-antitrypsin, because people with an inherited deficiency of this inhibitor are predisposed to pulmonary emphysema. The mechanism of lung destruction in these patients is still unclear but is believed to be due to protein-digesting enzymes produced by granulocytes and macrophages. These may cause emphysema even in people with normal levels of α_1-antitrypsin if they are released in excess by chronic lung irritation. It now looks as if pulmonary emphysema may be only one example of a degenerative disease where protein-digesting enzymes play a decisive role. For instance, one such enzyme, though of a type different from trypsin, has been found in the joints of patients with rheumatoid arthritis. Knowledge of the three-dimensional structure of these enzymes may open the way to the synthesis of tailor-made inhibitors for the treatment of such diseases.

HAEMOGLOBIN DISEASES

In 1949 Pauling, Itano, Singer and Wells published a paper entitled 'Sickle-cell anemia, a molecular disease'.[10] They showed that homozygotes suffering from this autosomal recessive disease had a haemoglobin which differed from the normal in that it lacked two negative charges. Ingram later discovered that this was due to a single amino acid residue among the 287 in the half molecule of haemoglobin being replaced: one glutamate was replaced by a valine. This was the first time that a genetic mutation was shown to cause the replacement of an amino acid in a protein.* A search for other haemoglobin diseases soon followed, and now over two hundred different abnormal haemoglobins are known, which give rise to a variety of haematological disorders whose cause had been unrecognized before; these may affect both the synthesis and the life span of red blood cells.

Haemoglobin consists of four haems and two pairs of protein chains called α and β. It transports oxygen from the lungs to the tissues and helps the return transport of carbon dioxide. This dual function depends on a reversible change of structure. The venous form of haemoglobin has a low affinity for oxygen and a high one for hydrogen ions, carbon dioxide and 2,3-diphosphoglycerate; in the arterial form these relative affinities are reversed. Efficient respiratory transport depends on correct regulation of the equilibrium between the two forms. My colleagues and I have determined their three-dimensional structure in atomic detail.[12,13] H. Lehmann and I then attempted to interpret the clinical symptoms of the haemoglobin diseases in stereochemical terms.[14] In most of them the abnormality consists of the replacement of a single amino acid residue, as it does in sickle cell anaemia, but the position of that residue is crucial in deciding the nature of the symptoms. If the residue lies on the surface, as often happens, there may not be any symptoms, at least in heterozygotes, because the haemoglobin molecule hardly 'feels' the wrong residue. In homozygotes, on the other hand, superficial replacements may reduce the solubility of the

---

* Recently the same replacement of a single glutamic acid by a valine has been found in a variant human α_1-antitrypsin (S). The replacement is harmless in heterozygotes (SM) carrying both the normal (M) and the variant (S) gene, but it may predispose SS homozygotes to pulmonary emphysema.[11]

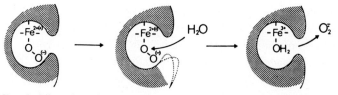

Fig. 5. Liberation of superoxide ion on autoxidation of haemoglobin. (Reproduced, with permission, from the article by Carrell *et al.*[16])

haemoglobin in the red cell. This happens in sickle cell anaemia where the venous form of haemoglobin actually crystallizes out. Prevention of this crystallization would relieve the disease, but has proved very difficult. The structure of the areas of contact between neighbouring molecules of sickle cell haemoglobin is now being worked out in atomic detail and may form the basis for a synthetic approach to the inhibition of crystallization.

The surface of the haemoglobin molecule is studded with electrically charged amino acid side chains which ensure its high solubility in water. Its interior structure, on the other hand, is stabilized by hydrocarbon side chains which make it impenetrable to water. In several abnormal haemoglobins this water-repellent armour is breached, so that they become unstable and form amorphous precipitates, known as Heinz bodies, in the red cell. Similar denatured precipitates are seen in thalassaemia where the red cells contain unequal numbers of α and β chains. The precipitates make the red cells more rigid and therefore more fragile, and this was believed to be the main cause of the associated haemolytic anaemias. Denaturation of haemoglobin is also accompanied by oxidation of the haem iron from its normal ferrous to the ferric state. It has now been found that it is this oxidation rather than the presence of denatured haemoglobin precipitates which mainly causes haemolysis. The mechanism is this. In the first step of the reaction the iron-bound oxygen molecule is reduced to superoxide ion which may then dissociate from the haem and produce hydrogen peroxide ion, hydroxyl radicals and singlet oxygen in the surrounding water (Fig. 5).[15] These are all oxidizing agents, hydroxyl radical being the most powerful among them, and they attack the lipids of the cell membrane, with resulting haemolysis. The obvious remedy is the administration of drugs, such as vitamin E or 2,3-dihydrobenzoic acid, that are designed to trap free radicals. These are now under trial.[16,17] In the long term practical results of much wider importance should result from the studies of the abnormal haemoglobins. In the first place those studies have shown that the genetic code in humans is the same as in *E. coli*, which is a prerequisite for relieving congenital diseases by any kind of genetic engineering. They have proved that human genes are subject to a fairly high rate of mutation (the frequency of abnormal haemoglobins in the human population may be greater than 1 in 500), but that these mutations may be harmless if they merely replace residues at the surface of enzymes away from their active sites. Interior replacements on the other hand, may affect the function and stability of enzymes. In favourable circumstances knowledge of their three-dimensional structure may allow us to mitigate such effects.

I started to study haemoglobin by X-ray crystallography in 1937 because at that time the structure of proteins seemed the most important unsolved problem in biochemistry, but I never dreamed that its solution would one day throw light on the nature of inherited diseases or would help to relieve them.

XERODERMA PIGMENTOSUM

The mutations which give rise to the abnormal haemoglobins occur spontaneously, perhaps by random errors inherent in the genetic process. It had long been known that the rate of mutation can be enhanced by external factors such as radiation and certain chemicals. It had also been suspected that some of the same factors which produce mutations give rise to cancer, but no exact correlation had been shown.

Ultraviolet light (u.v.) damages DNA by causing two pyrimidine bases—usually, but not always, on the same strand—to become covalently linked. In u.v.-sensitive bacteria this linkage inhibits DNA replication and thereby stops further growth. But there are strains of the same bacteria which are resistant to u.v. and it turns out that these possess an enzyme system which excises the dimers and repairs the gap, thus allowing growth to resume.[18] Now, it appears that normal human skin cells have an enzyme system for the repair of u.v. damage similar to that of u.v.-resistant bacteria. There is a rare autosomal recessive human disease in which the skin is extremely sensitive to u.v. light; it is called *xeroderma pigmentosum*. Sufferers from this disease—the homozygotes—are also very liable to skin cancer. In 1969 J. E. Cleaver discovered that fibroblasts from such patients lack the ability to repair u.v. damaged DNA.[19] Dutch investigators later found that there are six genetically distinct types of enzymic deficiency, that is, six complementation groups,[20] but Japanese workers have shown that u.v. resistance can be restored to five of the six types of fibroblasts by an enzyme which is an endonuclease from *E. coli* infected with T4 phage (Figs. 6 & 7).[21] Their results are exciting because they suggest that it may become possible to treat patients with this kind of enzyme, even if it is not yet clear how it could be applied.

DETECTION OF CHEMICAL CARCINOGENS

Discovery of the cause of *xeroderma pigmentosum* was important because it

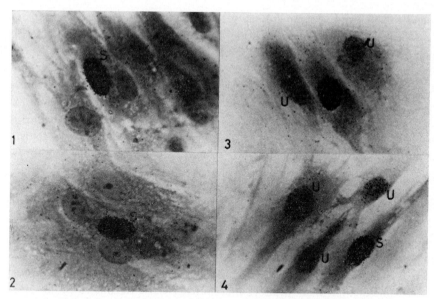

FIG. 6. Restoration of u.v.-induced 'unscheduled' (not connected with cell division) DNA synthesis of *Xeroderma pigmentosum* skin fibroblasts by treatment with T4 phage endonuclease (ENase). U.v.-inactivated Sendai virus (HVJ) is added to make the cells permeable to the enzyme. The pictures are autoradiograms showing the incorporation of [³H]thymidine into the cell nuclei. The cells were first u.v. irradiated, then treated with enzyme alone (1), or with HVJ alone (2), or with both the enzyme and HVJ (3), and then incubated with [³H]thymidine for three hours. For comparison, normal fibroblasts were u.v. irradiated, treated with HVJ alone and then incubated with [³H]thymidine for three hours (4). S marks cells heavily labelled in S phase. U marks lightly labelled cells showing unscheduled DNA synthesis. (Reproduced, with permission, from Tanaka *et al.*[21])

linked the occurrence of a cancer with a mutagenic event whose nature and repair could be explained in the same molecular terms as in bacteria. Evidence in favour of a causal link between the frequency of somatic mutation and the incidence of cancer has long been accumulating, yet many of the most potent chemical carcinogens seemed to have no mutagenic effect in microorganisms. This paradox was finally resolved by Bruce Ames, a molecular biologist. Ames had devoted nearly twenty years to the study of the control of protein synthesis in *Salmonella typhimurium*. His work, like that of Hartley and Blow's on chymotrypsin and mine on haemoglobin, was undertaken without any fore-knowledge of possible applications.

The chromosome of *Salmonella* contains a row of genes that code for the enzymes needed to make the amino acid histidine. Transcription of these genes into messenger RNA is controlled by a gene known as the operator which responds to the level of histidine in the cell, switching transcription on when

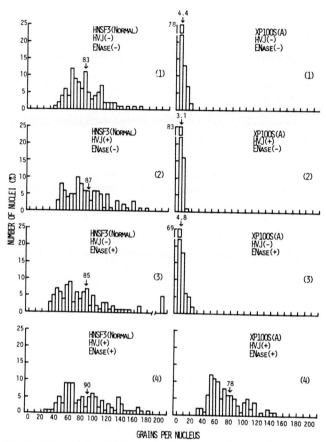

Fig. 7. Histograms showing numbers of silver grains produced by the disintegration of ³H labels after u.v. irradiation in nuclei of normal skin fibroblasts (left) and fibroblasts from a *xeroderma pigmentosum* patient (right). Conditions and abbreviations as in the legend for Fig. 6. (Reproduced, with permission, from Tanaka *et al.*[21])

histidine is scarce and switching it off when it is plentiful. Certain mutant strains of *Salmonella* cannot grow unless histidine is supplied in the medium; this has turned out to be due to mutations in the genes of the histidine operon. Ames decided to make use of the large number of available histidine mutants to develop a test for chemical mutagens. After screening hundreds of histidine mutants against known mutagens he selected four such strains. In one of them the DNA differs from that of the wild type in having an AT pair replaced by a GC pair, or vice versa. In the remaining three strains the DNA carries mutations of a kind first correctly interpreted by Crick, Barnett, Brenner and Watts-Tobin when they established the nature of the genetic code.[22,23] They showed

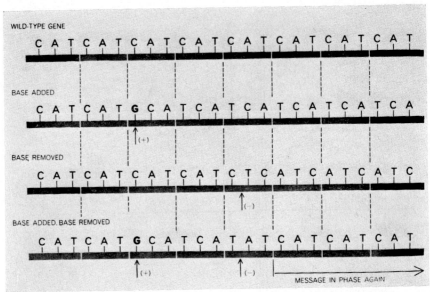

FIG. 8. The effect of mutations that add or remove a base is to shift the reading of the genetic message, assuming that the reading begins at the left-hand side of the gene. The hypothetical message in the wild-type gene is CAT,CAT... Adding a base shifts the reading to TCA, TCA... Removing a base makes it ATC, ATC... Addition and removal of a base puts the message in phase again. (Reproduced, with permission, from Crick.[23])

that a triplet of bases along a chain of nucleic acid codes for each amino acid residue along a protein chain (Fig. 8). The genetic code is read in sequence, so that the sequence of nucleotide bases makes sense only if the reading frame is positioned correctly with respect to the succession of coding triplets. Certain mutagens such as proflavine intercalate between the base pairs of DNA and thereby interfere with its replication so that base pairs are either added or deleted. If the number of base pairs added or deleted is not equal to three or a multiple of three, then the reading frame is shifted and the coding triplets that follow the site of mutation no longer make sense. Three of the four strains of *Salmonella* used by Ames carry mutations of this type in the histidine genes.[24,25] Ames plated these histidine-requiring strains of *Salmonella* on a histidine-free nutrient, applied chemical carcinogens and waited for the growth of colonies in which a reversion of the original mutation had allowed histidine biosynthesis to be resumed. The presence of 10^9 organisms on each plate allowed rare genetic events to be detected. The smallness of the bacterial chromosomes increased the likelihood of reversions of the original mutation as compared to other mutations which might be lethal. The time needed for one experiment was only two days.

Initially only some of the known chemical carcinogens caused growth of revertant colonies but Ames and his colleagues improved the sensitivity of his system step by step until he was able to prove a strong correlation between carcinogenicity and reversion. He introduced two additional mutations: one raises the sensitivity by eliminating the repair mechanism, already mentioned, that repairs u.v. and other damage, and the other strips the bacterial surface of part of its protective lipopolysaccharide layer which makes it more permeable to large molecules. He also increased mutagenesis in his tester strains by incorporating a plasmid which appears to channel DNA damage down an error-prone repair pathway (SOS repair).

Ames made one more improvement in the system which proved decisive. It had been discovered that in mammals many compounds are non-carcinogenic as such, but are converted into carcinogens by hydroxylating enzymes in the liver. Ames decided to mimic this conversion by adding rat or human liver homogenate together with a generating system for nicotinamide-adenine dinucleotide phosphate to his cultures. The results show a strong correlation between carcinogenesis in mammals and mutagenesis in *Salmonella*.[26,27] Ninety per cent (157/175) of the carcinogens were mutagenic in the test, including

TABLE 1

Correlation between carcinogenic (car) and mutagenic (mut) activity of chemicals

	car + mut +	car 0 mut 0	car + mut 0	car 0 mut +	?	% correlation
Aromatic amines etc.	21	9	2	–	12	94
Fungal toxins & antibiotics	8	2	–	2	2	83
Esters, epoxides, carbamates, etc.	14	6	4	2	2	77
Nitro aromatics & heterocycles	26	1	–	3	2	90
Miscellaneous heterocycles	1	7	3	–	–	73
Miscellaneous nitrogen compounds	7	2	2	2	–	69
Nitrosamines etc.	20	2	1	–	–	96
Polycyclic aromatics	27	7	–	3	1	92
Miscellaneous aliphatics & aromatics	1	10	4	–	5	73
Alkyl halides	16	1	3	2	2	77
Azo dyes & diazo compounds	12	2	–	1	2	93
Cigarette smoke condensate	1	–	–	–	–	100
Common biochemicals		42				100
Totals	154	91	19	15	28	88

106 Non-carcinogens { 14% positive, but / 86% negative   173 Carcinogens { 89% positive / 11% negative

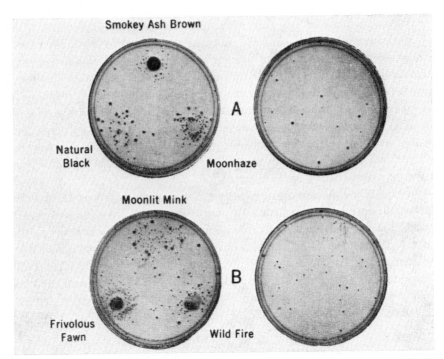

Fɪɢ. 9. Spot tests on Petri plates showing the mutagenicity of various hair dyes on a histidine-requiring strain of *Salmonella*. The spots are colonies which have regained the ability to make histidine by reversion of the original frame-shift mutation. (Reproduced, with permission, from Ames *et al.*[28])

almost all of the known human carcinogens that were tested. Despite the severe limitations inherent in defining non-carcinogenicity, few 'non-carcinogens' showed any degree of mutagenicity (Table 1). The mutagens include tar from cigarette smoke and oxidative hair dyes (Figs. 9, 10).[28] The latter discovery was alarming since twenty million women dye their hair in the US alone. Another mutagen is chloracetaldehyde, a possible metabolite of dichloroethane and of vinylchloride, two chemicals of which several million tons are produced in the US each year.

Ames's method offers a cheap, quick and sensitive way of screening chemicals for mutagenicity. For instance, 1 nanogram of 2-aminoanthracene doubled the spontaneous reversion rate of about twenty colonies, and 500 ng gave 11 000 revertant colonies compared to about thirty in the controls. In view of the correlation between mutagens and carcinogens any compound which is a potent mutagen is now suspected of also being carcinogenic.

The first impact of Ames's work should be the elimination of known carcino-

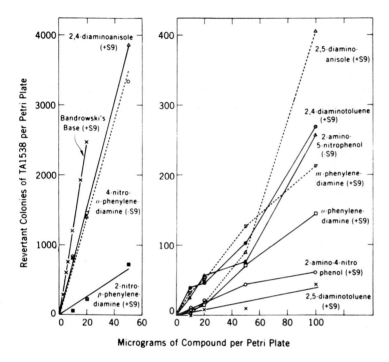

FIG. 10. Dose–response curves of the mutagenicity of chemicals extracted from hair dyes. Revertant colonies were counted after incubating the Petri plates for 48 hours at 37 °C with the chemical mutagen and the microsomal activation system (S9) where indicated. (Reproduced, with permission, from Ames *et al.*[28])

gens from our food and daily habits so that the number of carcinogenic events to which we are being exposed is reduced—and, incidentally, so that we can stop worrying about many other commonly used chemicals when they turn out to be harmless. In the long run this research and the work on *xeroderma pigmentosum* may help us to unravel the exact molecular mechanism by which u.v. irradiation and chemicals that revert frame shift and other mutations cause cancer.

What has molecular biology contributed to this work? It has supplied the basic concepts of microbial genetics, mutagenesis, repair and feedback control; and it has supplied the techniques of transferring genetic material from one strain of bacteria to another which Ames used to build up the sensitivity of his system. These concepts and techniques were developed by scientists who set out to interpret fundamental biological processes in physical and chemical terms. Generally the problems were so complex that it took many years to solve them. At the outset our ignorance was too profound for us to foresee the relation of our work to human disease. The relation became apparent only afterwards. Although we know more now than when we started, molecular biology is still too young a science for us to know exactly where it will pay off; hence we may do best if we spread our efforts over a wide field. Since research is the art of the soluble, it is often more profitable to study a basic problem in microorganisms where it can be solved, rather than in mammalian cells which are so much more complex. One of my examples has shown how such an indirect approach has helped to unravel pathogenic events in man. It would be a mistake if all molecular biologists switched to mammalian cells, as has recently become the fashion, or as they are being forced to do by policy decisions of supporting agencies. There is a unity of life at the molecular level which implies that anything found to be true in *E. coli* may also hold in man.

In the future, the most important contribution of molecular biology to medical practice may well be genetic engineering. Deliberate alteration of the human genome may remain in the realm of science fiction, but cheap manufacture of human proteins such as insulin, clotting factors or inhibitors of protein-digesting enzymes could lead to the relief of much suffering.

Discussion

Black: Molecular biology has great power in relation to the systems of the body and it is quite clearly an inexhaustible area of enquiry.

Perutz: I could not find an example of someone in molecular biology being given a million dollars and promptly solving a medically relevant problem. But in pharmacology, where relevant problems and the ways of attacking them are clearer, this seems to have happened. A natural morphine agonist in the brain was recently discovered, isolated and chemically synthesized as a result of funds having been made available for research on drug addiction by the National Institutes of Health and the Medical Research Council.[29] Similarly the exciting discovery that antipsychotic drugs react with and block the receptors for dopamine seems to have been made as a result of increased funds having been made available for research on mental disorder.[30]

Eisenberg: I suspect that the last phase in the enkephalin story was indeed a moment in history when a sufficiency of funds could have speeded up a process that followed after the previous five years of exploratory work. Liberal funding a decade earlier might not have altered that particular timetable.

Black: There seems to be a difference between finding out what is antagonizing or mopping up morphine in the brain, and finding out what causes cancer.

The problems seem to be of a different order. I would think that crash funding was appropriate to the first and not to the other.

Burgen: That is only half the enkephalin story, which is in a way a delayed logical story. It was known, of course, that morphine acted on the brain and is localized there. In the last few years workers in Sweden, the USA and the UK have shown that morphine binds specifically to parts of the brain and to membrane fractions from brain. The question was also asked why there was a morphine receptor in the brain and whether it has a normal function. It couldn't be just an accident of nature: nature doesn't have that kind of accident. The question was first asked about ten years ago, unfortunately in the wrong way. The structure of morphine had been known since 1925 and it was asked what natural compounds were known that are like morphine. The natural compounds seemed to be steroids, so steroids that would antagonize morphine were looked for but none were found. Then the empirical approach came back and extracts of brain were tested to see if they antagonized morphine. This was successful and isolation of the material and elucidation of its structure soon followed. The substance turned out to be a simple pentapeptide. This discovery promises an entirely new approach to the study of addiction and tolerance to opioids.[31]

Hiatt: We have heard today an exciting summary of what I am sure is just the beginning of the application of molecular biology to our understanding of disease. But can we bring fundamental and applied research even closer together? Bruce Ames says that he decided to explore the usefulness of *Salmonella* mutants in the mid-60s shortly after his four-year-old child brought him a packet of potato crisps to open. When he looked at the contents listed on the packet he found not only potatoes but several other compounds as well. In the library he could find very little information about those other compounds and what they might do to his child. He looked at available methodology for exploring carcinogenesis and mutagenesis and found this unsatisfactory. That was when he conceived of the possibility of using his mutants as the basis for testing chemicals for mutagenic activity. It is interesting to speculate whether we would even now have such a test, had Ames been childless.

Berliner: One of the most powerful mutagens that Ames was working on at the National Institutes of Health was caffeine.

Phillips: It may be worth reminding ourselves that most of us here were undergraduates before it was generally recognized that genes were nucleic acids, and certainly before it was worked out how these nucleic acids control the synthesis of proteins. As Dr Perutz says, molecular biology is really a very new subject, and we are supervising the education of people against a background of knowledge which wasn't available when we were educated ourselves.

That leads me to speculate that perhaps it isn't surprising that it is difficult to get this new information accepted and working as the basis of medicine. It is rather like an activation energy hump which one has to get over before the rapid take-off to a new higher level is possible.

During the period when new information has to be assimilated, the public image of medicine might even suffer from the availability of that information. For example, in 1950, before Dr Perutz had looked at abnormal haemoglobins, patients suffering from, say, haemoglobin M might have had what was to them better and more comforting general medical treatment than they might get now. Now they might simply be told there was no hope, that it was a genetic situation.

Perutz: A haematologist friend told me of an anaemic patient who had spent much money on investigations of her trouble in numerous haematology clinics. My friend discovered that the patient was a heterozygote for an abnormal haemoglobin and he told her that her condition was not likely to deteriorate. This put her mind at rest. So it helped to have the correct diagnosis even if there was no treatment.

References

1 HARTLEY, B. S. (1973) Homologies in serine proteinases. *Philosophical Transactions of the Royal Society of London B 257*, 77-86
2 BIRKTOFT, J. J., BLOW, D. M., HENDERSON, R. & STEITZ, T. A. (1973) The structure of α-chymotrypsin. *Philosophical Transactions of the Royal Society of London B 257*, 67-76
3 STROUD, R. M. (1974) A family of protein-cutting proteins. *Scientific American 231*, 74-89
4 BLOW, D. M. & SMITH, J. M. (1975) Enzyme substrate and inhibitor interactions. *Philosophical Transactions of the Royal Society of London B 272*, 87-98
5 HUBER, R., KUKLA, D., STEIGEMANN, W., DEISENHOFER, J. & JONES, A. (1974) Structure of the complex formed by bovine trypsin and bovine pancreatic trypsin inhibitor, in *Bayer Symposium V: Proteinase Inhibitors* (Fritz, H., *et al.*, eds.), pp. 497-512, Springer, Berlin
6 DAVIE, E. W. & KIRBY, E. P. (1973) Molecular mechanisms in blood coagulation. *Current Topics in Cellular Regulation 7*, 51-86
7 MAGNUSSON, S. (1975) The primary structure of prothrombin, the role of vitamin K in blood coagulation, and a thrombin-catalyzed 'negative feed-back' control mechanism for limiting the activation of prothrombin [and other papers in the same volume], in *Boerhaave Series for Postgraduate Medical Education* No. 10, pp. 25-46, Leiden University Press, Leiden
8 HAUSCHKA, P. V., LIAN, J. B. & GALLOP, P. M. (1975) Direct identification of the calcium-binding amino acid, γ-carboxylglutamate, in mineralized tissue. *Proceedings of the National Academy of Sciences of the USA 72*, 3925-3929
9 MARCINAC, E., FARLEY, C. H. & DeSIMONE, P. A. (1974) Familial thrombosis due to antithrombin III deficiency. *Blood 43*, 219-231
10 PAULING, L., ITANO, M. A., SINGER, S. J. & WELLS, I. C. (1949) Sickle-cell anemia, a molecular disease. *Science (Washington. D.C.), 110*, 543-548
11 OWEN, M. C. & CARRELL, R. W. (1976) Alpha-1-antitrypsin: molecular abnormality of S-variant. *British Medical Journal 1*, 130-131
12 PERUTZ, M. F. (1969) The haemoglobin molecule. *Proceedings of the Royal Society of London B 173*, 113-140

[13] FERMI, G. (1975) Three-dimensional Fourier synthesis of human deoxyhaemoglobin at 2.5 Å resolution: refinement of the atomic model. *Journal of Molecular Biology 97*, 237-256

[14] PERUTZ, M. F. & LEHMANN, H. (1968) Molecular pathology of human haemoglobin. *Nature (London), 219*, 902-909

[15] MISRA, H. P. & FRIDOVICH, I. (1972) The generation of superoxide radical during the autoxidation of haemoglobin. *Journal of Biological Chemistry 247*, 6960-6962

[16] CARRELL, R. W., WINTERBOURN, C. C. & RACHMILEWITZ, E. A. (1975) Activated oxygen and haemolysis. *British Journal of Haematology, 30*, 259-264

[17] GRAZIANO, J. H., GRADY, R. W. & CERAMI, A. (1975) The identification of 2,3-dihydro-benzoic acid as a potentially useful iron-chelating drug. *Journal of Pharmacology and Experimental Therapeutics, 190*, 570-575

[18] SETLOW, R. B. & CARRIER, W. L. (1964) The disappearance of thymine dimers from DNA: an error-correcting mechanism. *Proceedings of the National Academy of Sciences of the USA 51*, 226-231

[19] CLEAVER, J. E. (1969) Xeroderma pigmentosum: a human disease in which an initial stage of DNA repair is defective. *Proceedings of the National Academy of Sciences of the USA 63*, 428-435

[20] KRAEMER, K. H., COON, H. G., PETINGA, R. A., BARRETT, S. F., RAHE, A. E. & ROBBINS J. H. (1975) Genetic heterogeneity in *xeroderma pigmentosum*: complementation groups and their relationship to DNA repair rates. *Proceedings of the National Academy of Sciences of the USA 72*, 59-63

[21] TANAKA, K., SEKIGUCHI, M. & OKADA, Y. (1975) Restoration of ultraviolet-induced unscheduled DNA synthesis of *xeroderma pigmentosum* cells by the concomitant treatment with bacteriophage T4 endonuclease V and HVJ (Sendai virus). *Proceedings of the National Academy of Sciences of the USA 72*, 4071-4075

[22] CRICK, F. H. C., BARNETT, L., BRENNER, S. & WATTS-TOBIN, R. J. (1961) General nature of genetic code for proteins. *Nature (London) 192*, 1227-1232

[23] CRICK, F. H. C. (1962) The genetic code. *Scientific American 207*, 66-73

[24] AMES, B. N. (1971) in *Chemical Mutagens: Principles and Methods for their Detection* (Hollaender, A., ed.) vol. 1, pp. 267-282, Plenum Press, New York

[25] AMES, B. N., GURNEY, E. G., MILLER, J. A. & BARTSCH, H. (1972) Carcinogens as frame-shift mutants. *Proc. Nat. Acad. Sci. US, 69*, 3128-3132

[26] McCANN, J., CHOI, E., YAMASAKI, E. & AMES, B. N. (1975) Detection of chemical carcinogens as mutagens in the Salmonella microsome test: assay of 300 chemicals. *Proceedings of the National Academy of Sciences of the USA 72*, 5135-5139

[27] McCANN, J. & AMES, B. N. (1976) Detection of chemical carcinogens as mutagens in the Salmonella microsome test: assay of 300 chemicals. Part II. *Proceedings of the National Academy of Sciences of the USA 73*, 950-954

[28] AMES, B. N., KAMMEN, H. O. & YAMASAKI, E. (1975) Hairdyes are mutagenic. *Proceedings of the National Academy of Sciences of the USA 72*, 2423-2427

[29] SNYDER, S. H. (1975) Opiate receptor in normal and drug altered brain function. *Nature (London) 257*, 185-189

[30] IVERSON, L. L. (1975) Dopamine receptors in the brain. *Science (Washington, D.C.) 188*, 1084-1089

[31] HUGHES, J., SMITH, T. W., KOSTERLITZ, H. W., FOTHERGILL, L. A., MORGAN, B. A. & MORRIS, H. R. (1975) Identification of two related pentapeptides from the brain with potent opiate agonist activity. *Nature (London) 258*, 577-579

French medical research:
the risk of 'demedicalization'

PHILIPPE MEYER

INSERM U7, Hopital Necker, Paris

Abstract   French medical research is at present financed almost entirely by INSERM (Institut National de la Santé et de la Recherche Médicale). The INSERM budget (286 million francs in 1975) supports research in laboratories in university hospitals by doctors who have both clinical and teaching commitments and, especially, by more than a thousand 'statutory research workers' employed by INSERM.

Research in INSERM laboratories now tends to be fundamental biological research rather than directed towards pathological problems. Among the reasons for this are (*i*) the mode of recruitment of statutory research workers; (*ii*) the difficulties of clinical investigation, which are due mainly to the way the hospitals function and to lack of interest by the hospital administration in medical research; (*iii*) the small number of university doctors actively involved in research.

Research on fundamental biological problems in INSERM laboratories is making excellent progress, due to the quality of the research workers, and it may pay in the long run. But medical research is now tending to become an 'ivory tower' for the victorious researchers, who sometimes scorn the clinicians.

Medical research will, if no measures are taken, 'demedicalize'. Institutes of pure biological research could soon be isolated within the medical faculties and doctors may become even less scientific and investigative than they are today. This situation could be modified by: (*i*) re-evaluating the role of research in a university hospital career, making it impossible for a doctor to attain high levels of promotion unless he does some research (this could be done by asking doctors interested in such a career to work for several years in an INSERM laboratory after their training and before they take up clinical responsibilities); (*ii*) awarding clinicians, exceptionally, the status of research worker; (*iii*) increasing considerably the participation of the universities in financing medical research, a participation which at present is absurdly low and is ever decreasing.

The fundamental goal of all research undertaken by man is absolute progress in knowledge. In this task he is without doubt motivated by an existential anxiety that is due to the unknown which surrounds him. Research undertaken by physicians or certain biologists interested in human health is motivated, above all, by one specific preoccupation, the essence of which is to improve the condition of the sick.

Neglect or omission of this superior objective in the dynamics of a piece of research assigns it to the category of pure biological research as opposed to medical research. Of course, such pure biological research, since it concerns living matter, can contribute essential information to the understanding of the function or disorder of human life processes. But the time lapse before any progress in human health is achieved is long, and the means by which the results are integrated with such progress are often devious.

The bodies responsible for medical research in France have been remarkably efficient in accomplishing its 'renaissance'. However, the very nature of these bodies and their relationship with those responsible for the development of medicine are such that they now seem to us to compromise their objective. This article analyses the causes and the consequences of this phenomenon and suggests remedial measures.

DEVELOPMENT OF THE STRUCTURE OF FRENCH MEDICAL RESEARCH

The situation in France between the two World Wars was not favourable to medical research. Apart from work at the Institut Pasteur (whose quality was by far inferior to that performed at the time of its creation) and in the Collège de France, and the restricted research subsidized by the Centre National de la Recherche Scientifique (CNRS), research was practically absent from the French medical scene. This lethargy continued until the years 1950–1960, during which a few adventurous physicians, fired by studies undertaken in the Anglo-Saxon community, managed to impart their enthusiasm to certain benevolent and enlightened politicians. A shadow institute without proper funding, the Institut National d'Hygiène, had been created during the Second World War for the study of public health problems. After the war, this institute financed an embryonic research programme until 1964, when the organization underwent a metamorphosis into the Institut National de la Santé et de la Recherche Médicale (INSERM). This 19-year time lag between the end of the Second World War and the creation of INSERM is indeed distressing but it merits exposure since it reflects the viscosity of the administration and the difficulties that physicians avid to perform research encountered in making themselves heard by the government and by their colleagues—who were, by tradition, little inclined to follow them.

The slow and difficult birth of INSERM has not, however, compromised its development, which has rapidly become explosive, with INSERM now the principal, if not the only organization subsidizing French medical research.

In principle, French medical research is financed by five public organizations and one private body, the Fondation pour la Recherche Médicale Française. The functioning of this last body is hazardous, since it depends on the generosity of individuals. The five public organizations are INSERM, the universities, the Délégation Générale à la Recherche Scientifique et Technique (DGRST), the CNRS and the Association Claude-Bernard.[1] The contribution of the university is absurdly low, the money distributed being scarcely enough to finance practical teaching, which has become difficult because of the vast numbers of students, and it cannot practically support any useful research. The few university doctors with research activities are obliged to rely on funds from other organizations. The DGRST has considerable budgetary resources but these are destined for specific research projects considered of prime importance by the government technical advisers. The financial means of the CNRS are also considerable but they cover a large number of research activities, among which medical research is rather low on the priority list. Most of its funds support costly research in physics and chemistry. The budget of the Association Claude-Bernard is supplied by the Ville de Paris and hence finances only certain particularly dynamic hospital departments in Paris.

The predominance of INSERM suggested by the above analysis is further illustrated by what follows. Since its creation in 1964, INSERM has financed the construction of 74 laboratories, called 'Unités de Recherche' (research units), whose buildings and equipment have recently been reviewed with praise,[2] and it has equipped other laboratories made available under contract by various universities and public hospitals, permitting the installation of 55 'Groupes de Recherche' (research teams). In 1975 the annual budget of INSERM, supplied almost entirely by the Ministry of Public Health, reached 286.5 million francs (over £ 30 million), covering the running costs of research and the salaries of 1064 research workers and 1849 engineers, technicians and administrators.

These 1064 research workers do full-time research and do not participate in either teaching or clinical medicine. Their career progresses via the grades of 'Stagiaire', 'Attaché', 'Chargé' and 'Maître', to finish, for the more fortunate, as 'Directeur de Recherches'. In the grades of Stagiaire and Attaché people may be dismissed if their work proves to be unsatisfactory, but this occurs rarely. Once the grade of Chargé de Recherches is reached, the researcher is assured of a permanent position until the age of sixty-five years, his subsequent progression theoretically depending on his efforts and results. This position of full-time research worker is not unique to INSERM; CNRS personnel (of whom a minority interested in medical research work in INSERM laboratories) also have a similar status.

Working alongside these statutory research workers in the INSERM research units are university hospital doctors: 'Internes des Hôpitaux', 'Chefs de Clinique–Assistants des Hôpitaux', 'Maîtres de conférences agrégés' and 'Professeurs'. All have considerable teaching or clinical commitments, or both, which obviously restricts the time available for their research. The direction of units or research teams in INSERM may be undertaken by either statutory research workers or university hospital doctors. Directors are nominated for a five-year period, renewable if recommended by the Scientific Council of INSERM.

PROBLEMS ARISING IN MEDICAL RESEARCH: ORIGIN OF ITS 'DEMEDICALIZATION'

The INSERM statutory research workers used to be trained in the medical faculties (which in France are quite separate from the science faculties). Some chose to carry out full-time research by vocation; others, unfortunately the majority, chose this career because a university hospital career appeared to them to be not easily accessible. In general, the quality of the newly recruited research workers was not high.

The mode of recruitment of statutory research workers was changed in 1968 with the aim of improving their quality. This modification resulted in the selective recruitment of either doctors carefully prepared for research by advanced scientific studies in France or abroad, or non-medical scientists, from the Faculté des Sciences or from the Ecoles d'Ingénieurs.

The quality of the research achieved in INSERM laboratories gained much from this reform. For the last three or four years, candidates from the Faculté des Sciences have been preferentially recruited as research workers over candidates from the Faculté de Médecine. This practice does not, of course, compromise the level of research but does appear to lead to serious risks of eventual demedicalization, in the sense described above. Several factors appear to contribute to such an evolution. The first concerns the financial position of statutory research workers compared to that of university hospital doctors. The salaries of the former are inferior to those of the latter since statutory research workers do not receive the extra salary which the hospital administration pays to all university hospital doctors. This difference in salary, minimal to begin with, becomes very marked at higher levels of the university hospital career (Maître de conférences agrégé and Professeur). This inequality is obviously the source of delicate psychological problems arising between personnel working together in the same laboratory. For this reason also, young doctors are more tempted by a university hospital career than by that of a statutory research worker. Without doubt a university hospital career has become more difficult today because too few posts are available for recruitment. But this has not favoured an influx of doctors into an INSERM career, since many of them, realizing their slender chances in a university hospital career, orient themselves towards general practice which still remains relatively lucrative.

The second factor results from the position of most doctors *vis-à-vis* INSERM. The number of university doctors truly interested in research is still very small and this is not one of the criteria considered for the recruitment of Maître de conférences agrégé and Professeur. One may say without exaggeration that access to these high-ranking university posts is determined only by the number of posts allotted by the administration to each department, this itself being directly a function of the importance of the clinical activity of the department. The number of posts for Maître de conférences agrégé and Professeur in a department never exceeds three. For this reason, a Chef de Clinique desiring to reach this level chooses to make his career in a department where the number of such posts already filled is less than three. His success will then be only a function of his qualities in clinical medicine and his willingness to teach. His research activities are usually not considered, since the director of the department is usually not interested. Two factors thus appear to be responsible for the rift between the medical faculties and INSERM: on the one hand the lack of interest of most university doctors in research, and on the other, the lack of interest in research of most medical candidates, the latter factor of course being determined by the former. Thirdly, the influx of personnel with a purely scientific background into INSERM is due to the structure of non-medical scientific education in France. This type of education is undertaken both by the Faculté des Sciences, whose high educational quality in certain fields is put at risk by an excessive number of students, and by the Grandes Ecoles, which assure their pupils of an education whose adaptation to current problems is debatable but which has the advantage of being lavish for the students, who are selected for admission by a 'concours' (competitive examination). The reputation of the Grandes Ecoles, which is higher than that of the Faculté des Sciences, ensures that their pupils obtain important posts, the number of students trained in these schools corresponding roughly to the needs of French industrial activity. Many qualified students from the Faculté des Sciences certainly reach INSERM laboratories with a sincere inclination towards research, but in many cases material considerations also play a role. Science students are, in fact, often less fortunate than their colleagues trained in the Grandes Ecoles in the search for employment. Their numerous applications for posts at INSERM reflect this present predicament.

A fourth factor contributing to the tendency of INSERM research labora-

TABLE 1

Numbers of statutory research workers from two fields of medicine working at different levels in INSERM[3]

	Field			
	Reproduction		Nephrology, cardiology and respiration	
	INSERM statutory research workers (total no.)	INSERM statutory research workers (total no. of medical origin)	INSERM statutory research workers (total no.)	INSERM statutory research workers (total no. of medical origin)
Directeurs & Maîtres de Recherche	27	23	27	24
Chargés de Recherche	60	30	55	35
Attachés & Stagiaires	48	30	58	19

tories to become demedicalized is related to the quality of the scientific achievements in the last few years. The mode of recruitment of research workers, described above, has led to research carried out predominantly at the molecular level. The reputation of clinical investigation has thus suffered and this type of research has tended to be abandoned both by the central administrative bodies advising on research options, and by the research workers themselves.

Two examples illustrating the small number of statutory research workers of medical origin at present employed in certain sectors of INSERM are given in Table 1. It is clear that the percentage of personnel with a medical background is lowest in the rank of Attaché, i.e. among the most recently recruited.

The dynamism of certain INSERM research workers—together with the increasing multiplicity of occupations which prevent ageing university hospital doctors whose positions are not renewed from performing research—naturally results in the laboratories being run more and more by the statutory research workers, who are often of non-medical origin. One can thus predict that in the not-too-distant future the research units of INSERM will be directed by research workers whose only medical background, in certain cases, comes from their professional coexistence with medical men. The phenomenon of demedicalization will thus reach a maximum, since it is difficult to imagine how dialogue can persist between directors of research laboratories and neighbouring doctors overburdened with clinical and teaching duties, even if any friendship exists between them. INSERM thus runs the risk of becoming an institute comparable in its vocation to the CNRS, in spite of its laboratories being in hospitals.

SUGGESTED REMEDIES FOR THE DEMEDICALIZATION OF INSERM

The solutions proposed here are, in theory, fairly straightforward. However, if applied, they would solve many serious problems, since complete reshuffling of the medical and university bodies would be necessary.

The first measure proposed concerns the recruitment of the 'Maîtres de conférences agrégés' and 'Professeurs' of the Faculté de Médecine. I suggest a compulsory probation period of one or more years for the Chefs de clinique in INSERM laboratories, during which time they would carry out personally a research project under the control of the director of the laboratory. At the end of this period of research, whose duration would depend on the nature of the research undertaken, the doctor would have to choose between a university hospital career and that of a statutory research worker. The quality of the research performed would, of course, be one of the fundamental criteria in the selection of the Maîtres de conférences for the Conseils de Faculté. This measure would result in the production of medical doctors capable of carrying out medical research and also in the production of clinicians more highly trained than they are today in the analysis of illness and hence of its treatment.

The second measure concerns the research workers from the Faculté des Sciences recruited by INSERM. They too should have a choice between remaining in full-time research or joining the ranks of the basic science lecturers of the Faculté de Médecine, even though they lack a medical qualification. The former choice would maintain the fundamental approach to medical research which is so important today; the second, which runs against the present legislation reserving teaching posts for the medically qualified, would be useful in introducing personnel with advanced scientific backgrounds into the teaching ranks.

These two measures could be complemented by exchange possibilities between positions at high levels, that is between lecturers at the Faculté de Médecine and directors of research at INSERM. One can imagine that a lecturer would be happy to interrupt his teaching activities—temporarily, of course—to dedicate his time entirely to personal research, or to directing research carried out by a team who may need his direction. One can just as easily imagine that a director of research may want to teach and could then be admitted for a certain time into the teaching ranks.

The results of all these measures can be put schematically (Fig. 1). They would ensure that all kinds of competence, however acquired, would be

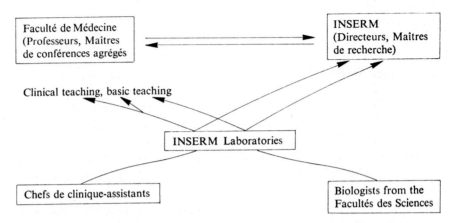

FIG. 1. Schematic remedies for demedicalization.

available within one system whose fundamental concern is the condition of the sick. These measures would, in my opinion, diminish the risks of demedicalization of research, since they abolish the barriers which exist between research laboratories and the Faculté de Médecine. They introduce a new concept, at least in the tradition of the French universities, of the task accomplished prevailing over the title of the person involved. These measures would in consequence reduce the risks of people growing old in positions which could become routine.

These diverse propositions in practice run up against many problems which must be solved before the reforms can be put into practice. Among the problems that may be mentioned are the disparity between salaries of university hospital doctors and university research workers, the harmful ascendancy of the diploma of Docteur en Médecine, the sectarianism of the Faculté de Médecine, the difficulties felt by the hospital administration in confiding research activities to personnel whom it considers by interest and tradition to be primarily clinicians, and the hostility of some statutory research workers who refuse, out of resentment due to their position, all dialogue with medical teachers. They will, of course, clash with the conservatism of most university hospital doctors who cannot grasp the necessity for research training before clinical activity.

I am conscious that the proposed reforms are too profound and radical to be enforced in their entirety. Single minor modifications, gradually enforced, would perhaps have a greater chance of success.

No matter what the consequences in France of these suggestions may be,

I hope that they may be useful to medical schools in other countries where there is a risk of similar errors being made.

ACKNOWLEDGEMENT

I wish to thank Mrs Mary J. Osborne-Pellegrin for her help with the manuscript.

Discussion

Black: As a former nephrologist I am very conscious of the great achievements of French medical research in many fields, which must represent a triumph over the system. Is there much support for your view that the system needs to be changed, Dr Meyer?

Meyer: Yes, some people are now actively considering the problem.

Querido: You say that the research system in France is *bad*, Dr Meyer, which in the context of our meeting means that it must have a harmful effect on medical practice. How could that be established with certainty? The problem is not unique to France and you have no strong case.

Meyer: It is difficult to answer that. The clinical departments associated with INSERM units are the best and therefore INSERM has helped greatly in improving the quality of medical teaching and probably that of medical practice.

Saracci: I wonder what fraction of health services expenditure the biomedical research budget in France represents? Table 1 tells a worrying story about Italy. The real amount of biomedical research expenditure is even less than indicated (around 0.03% of GNP and 0.4% of health services expenditure in

TABLE 1 (Saracci)

Biomedical research expenditure in Italy

Year	Dollars per head (at constant 1974 value)		Total as % of GNP	Total as % of health services expenditure
	Total	Public		
1965	1.40	1.14 (0.17)	0.08	2.2
1968	1.42	1.16 (0.23)	0.07	1.7
1971	1.74	1.49 (0.30)	0.07	1.1
1974	1.62	1.34 (0.22)	0.06	0.8

Figures in brackets represent the amount channelled through the National Research Council (main individual component of the public expenditure actually used for research).

1974) because the current method of accounting includes under 'research' the salaries of the university personnel whose time is in fact largely spent in teaching.

Fliedner: The European research systems are surprisingly different from each other. In Germany the major contribution for medical research comes from the Deutsche Forschungsgemeinschaft (DFG; German Research Society), which supports all types of research. Table 2 gives examples of its budget.[4]

TABLE 2   (Fliedner)

Research expenditure in Germany

	Total research budget	Theoretical & practical medicine	Biological research
	(Million DM)		
1965	139		
1970	289		
1972	451	83.9	39.9
1973	542	103.4	44.8
1974	594	106.9	47.5

The DFG therefore spends a large proportion of its money on theoretical and clinical medicine, and this is almost exclusively spent in the university hospitals.

In Germany full professors (H4), associate professors (H3) and assistant professors (H2) have tenure, that is lifelong employment in the civil service, but lecturers (H1) do not. To move from research associate (A13) to lecturer (H1), one has to present a thesis (summarizing one's work in the previous four to six years); and to move from lecturer to assistant professor one has to apply for positions on a competitive basis. Only those with the best *research* qualifications succeed in becoming professors. The others have to leave if they do not find a permanent position within the university system.

A lot of money is spent on this system where people have to compete for the leading positions on the basis of their research accomplishments. I have studied what fraction of the research done in university hospitals is actually supported by the DFG, taking leukaemia research as an example and seeing who presented papers on leukaemia at national and international scientific meetings. I was surprised to find that the DFG was supporting about 10% of the research on leukaemia being published in these various meetings. I presume the same may be true in other fields. This means that in the universities, much more research is being done than is being supported by the DFG. This is because in Germany all universities and all faculties of medicine are state-owned and the state provides the basic support for running a department, including some research. The difficulty in Germany is that the departments are established largely on the basis of the traditional disciplines of medicine. In other words, new developments have little chance of becoming recognized because they are not considered as important in training medical students. The state apparently does not consider it important to develop new areas, because the postgraduate aspect and the research aspect are not recognized as being important in the usual university setting. So we cannot establish new areas easily and the trend is for people to go into established areas where more positions are available.

Dollery: I was very impressed by the quality of the INSERM research units I saw in 1973. The deliberate policy of sending people for training abroad, mainly to the US, was working well but it led to two problems. One was that research was much stronger in basic sciences than in clinical subjects. This was because of the difficulty of getting clinical research going when most of the teachers were overwhelmed with clinical teaching, and because of the strong emphasis on private practice which still exists in France. The other problem was that INSERM had just given security of tenure to all except their most junior staff. Since most of the people were young, the INSERM administration were forecasting that recruitment in future would be very small. This is not just a French problem. In England the MRC has given security of tenure on much the same terms to its staff. What is to be done with the middle-aged or elderly research worker who is no longer very good but has tenure?

Black: About thirty years ago in the UK there was considerable lack of contact between clinical practice, uncontaminated by research, and full-time research, similar to the present system as described by Dr Meyer in France.

Berliner: It is interesting to hear that research is not a matter of interest to universities. The usual complaint in the US is exactly the opposite, that people are selected for their research and for nothing else.

Eisenberg: Since World War II every professorial choice in the US has been based, wisely or foolishly, on an assessment of either the quality or the quantity of papers produced, sometimes to the point of absurdity. It is striking to hear that quite the opposite happens in France.

Meyer: Yes, but it should be realized that I was giving a general picture. Research is still considered as the criterion of selection in some departments.

Eisenberg: I understand that in France people begin to acquire civil service tenure in a field like physics during their years as graduate students, so they get built into the university system well before they have had to prove themselves as competent investigators. That seems wrong for a research system.

Saracci: Security of job tenure and job mobility are to be seen as distinct problems. Jobs are to be guaranteed but mobility should be too. This is vital in research. The unfortunate dominant trend in Italy is to make people stick permanently to a career line through tenure given as early as possible and career compartmentalization: mobility between university, hospitals and research institutions (not to speak of industrial laboratories and civil service jobs) is becoming almost impossible.

Berliner: Our National Institutes of Health in the US has many of the same problems as INSERM. One problem NIH has not been able to solve is the discrepancy in salaries between medical people inside and outside the organization. As regards tenure, NIH hires people by the civil service method and in our civil service people have tenure after one year. The NIH, however, has devised a number of methods—fellowships etc.—for delaying civil service status for its scientists. They now take three to five years to acquire tenure in the civil service system, and are usually about thirty-two or thirty-three years old by then. This is still sooner than one would like but at least the acquisition of tenure is delayed a bit.

Randle: Aren't research workers in the US Public Health Service entitled to a pension after fifteen or twenty years' service, making them an attractive proposition for universities? Is this a way of creating turnover among full-time career research workers?

Berliner: People who are commissioned officers in the Public Health Service, like those in the armed forces, are eligible for retirement after twenty years. They can take another job perhaps in their middle or late forties. But the civil service requires many more years than that.

Black: I sometimes have a nightmare that medical students will get tenure....

Hiatt: How old are people who become professors in Germany?

Fliedner: For full professors in medical sciences the range is from thirty-seven to fifty-five years. Assistant professors are usually about thirty to forty years of age.

Randle: What is the success rate in transition from lecturer to assistant professor?

Fliedner: I have no data on that.

Hjort: On tenure, we have considered only the aspect of getting rid of people. The lesson is that since more people are trained in research than can become professors, alternative careers should be provided which those who do not become professors can accept without losing face. Such people are useful in administration, in public health and in clinical medicine, so we should provide alternative pathways. This question is more important for the non-clinically-trained people: if we invite them to help us in medical research, we must provide alternative careers when necessary.

Luft: We have a tenure problem in Sweden too. After six months in any profession people cannot be fired. In the medical profession we have been trying to get round this problem by setting up an educational programme for each doctor when he finishes his studies. He applies with that programme to a teaching hospital; and by law he has to leave the teaching hospital after finishing his programme and becoming a specialist or general physician. If we want to keep him in that hospital he gets a lifetime position. We do not know yet whether this will work.

In Sweden, as in the United States, what matters in applying for a chair of medicine is sometimes not the number but the weight of papers produced. That is all right for good research workers. The trouble is that most clinical research workers who have clinical experience stop doing research when they get their professorial chairs. Only a very few continue doing research after the age of fifty and this is harmful to medical research.

References

[1] BURG, C. (1973). The organization and support of biomedical research in France, in *Medical Research Systems in Europe (Ciba Foundation Symposium 21)*, pp. 68-75, Associated Scientific Publishers, Amsterdam

[2] DOLLERY, C. T. & BURN, J. I. (1973). Clinical medicine and research in France. *British Medical Journal 2*, 601-604

[3] INSERM (1975) Institut National de la Santé et de la Recherche Médicale, 10 ans. (Bureau des Relations avec la Presse de l'INSERM, ed.), Avenir Graphique, Paris

[4] Deutsche Forschungsgemeinschaft (1974) *Tätigkeitsbericht 1974* (Jahresbericht Band I)

Health services research: why and how?

PETER F. HJORT

Section for Haematology, Rikshospitalet, Oslo*

Abstract It is useful to divide medical research into three areas: biomedical, clinical, and health services research. The areas partly overlap, and health services research is also related to social services research.

Research is carried out to solve problems and is an instrument for change. Health services research has developed over the last ten years in response to increasing problems in many health services. Superficially, these problems are caused by insufficient resources, but no service can hope to pay its way out of them. Some may be fairly accurately investigated, like need, demand, and utilization of care. Others are more complicated, e.g. evaluation of care, defining standards, and cost–benefit analyses. A few deal with fundamental values, like quality of life and responsibility of individuals and societies.

So far, health services research has led to greater emphasis on primary care, but it is fair to say that it has not managed to infiltrate the service and influence people's attitudes and ambitions. In the future, one must bring health services research inside the service and involve the professionals more deeply. One must support prevention studies, attack the ethical and clinical problems related to quality of life, study the potential of non-professional support in the community, and promote rational attitudes among professions, patients, people and politicians. The task is never-ending and health services research, therefore, must be part of the programme of all medical schools.

For me to discuss health services research at a symposium in London is an alarming case of an egg talking to a group of very accomplished hens. I must therefore start with an apology and an explanation.

Based on long traditions in epidemiology, health services research has expanded rapidly over the last ten to fifteen years in the UK. Norway has had relatively more money per head for the health service and has just begun to realize that money cannot buy an unlimited service. Last summer, the medical

---

* *Present address*: Institutt for Almenmedisin, Oslo

151

branch of The Norwegian Research Council for Science and the Humanities realized that we had to develop health services research, and I spent eight weeks in the UK in autumn 1975 to assemble the general information we need to start a research group. My own qualifications are severely limited, since I have not. been trained in health services research. My background is clinical haematology and university administration, and I still think and feel as a clinician. My reasons for attempting to develop health services research are simple: I believe medicine has reached a point where we must accept that resources are limited, and doctors should help to work out solutions and policies.

In this presentation, I shall not review the present state of health services research, but rather attempt to clarify why we need this research and how I believe it should be organized.

DEFINITION OF HEALTH SERVICES RESEARCH

Let me first briefly define the subject. It is useful to divide medical research into three broad groups:
(1) Biomedical, dealing with mechanisms of diseases;
(2) Clinical, dealing with the clinical picture, diagnosis, therapy and prognosis of diseases;
(3) Health services research, dealing with the needs for and functioning of the health services.
The groups overlap, and research on prevention belongs in all groups. The division line between basic and applied research goes through the middle of the second group. These distinctions are, I believe, sufficiently clear to be useful, and there is no need for more rigid definitions.

It may help to have a visual model of health services research. Any health service has to balance supply against needs, and in an ideal society the two might conceivably be equal. However, concepts of health are relative and influenced by traditions, culture, expectations and many other things. Therefore, there is a constantly shifting, dynamic relationship:

$$\text{Needs} \quad \rightleftharpoons \quad \text{Supply}$$

Health services research may be seen as a sensing system interposed between the two, to monitor needs and services so that people's health and the health service they get can be improved.

WHY HEALTH SERVICES RESEARCH?

I now turn to the first question: why health services research? In general, research is done to solve problems, thereby increasing fundamental knowledge, improving practical work, or both. In applied research, practical improvements are the immediate goal, but good research aims in addition for general knowledge.

The proper answer to my question should therefore be a list of the problems of the health service, selected as being important, soluble, and not tackled by biomedical and clinical research. Such problems will vary from country to country, but the following list is valid for a western country with some form of national health service.

Needs

The first thing to find out is obviously the total need, the job in hand. This is a difficult task, because need is influenced by traditions, values and social conditions, by the doctors, and by the supply of services.[1] In addition, there is the iceberg of unfelt needs which may be uncovered by screening. To define needs, therefore, is not a simple epidemiological task. Some speak with despair of the bottomless pit of needs, others state more cynically that needs are simply equal to supply plus 10–20%. When services are being planned, however, one obviously must use some data to express needs, especially changes in need. In Norway, for example, the number of people who are seventy years old or more increases by about 8000 every year.

Constraints

The next problem lies in the constraints, and there are at least three. The first is obviously money, and many believe that this is the only problem. Most countries enjoyed a rapid growth of their health services after the war, but the growth is slowing down painfully in most countries. The second constraint is a lack of manpower, especially in the professional groups. There is of course a relation between money and manpower: if there is little money, there is more manpower, and vice versa. Together these constraints force us to balance one service and one life against another, to make extremely difficult choices, and to establish priorities. This requires some ideas of costs, effectiveness and benefits of alternatives, thus bringing economy into medicine. The third constraint is rarely mentioned. It has to do with human and social costs of advanced medicine, quality of life and similar ethical problems. These costs begin to emerge, for example for kidney failure[2] and spina bifida.[3] For the old these problems will increase, paradoxically, as we improve services. The problem may be illustrated by acute leukaemia in patients over sixty years of age. Their chances of remission are small and the chances of serious side effects are high. Furthermore, it is my feeling that the human costs are especially high in people who are poor in human and social resources. I believe that these problems will increase, and in the future the slogan may be: we can afford to do what is right, but we do not yet know what is right.

Diseases and disabilities

More and more we shall have to think in terms of groups of patients; for example:
What is the total problem of hypertension in the society? How should it be diagnosed and treated? What resources are required and what benefit can be expected?
What is a sensible programme for haemophilia?
How shall we deal with low back pain, its diagnosis and therapy?
This kind of thinking will be forced upon us not only by limited resources, but also by demands for equality, and the answers require extensive research of all three kinds mentioned above.

Service policies

Health services can be divided into three major components:
(1) Primary care or general practice;
(2) Hospitals, mainly for short-term investigations and treatment;
(3) Long-term care in hospitals and in the community.
Since the war, hospitals have increased their share of the total health budgets —in the UK, for instance, from 55% in 1950 to 66% in 1972.[1] However, increasing hospital costs appear to have reached a point of diminishing returns, and the other two components demand a better deal. The increased numbers of old people add weight to these claims, and —at least in theory— many health services want to shift their emphasis from the hospitals to the communities. This has proved very difficult. The hospitals are here and must be run and kept up. They are large and powerful institutions and, furthermore, they are often the largest employers in the cities. Changes are therefore bitterly fought, and many politicians have been humiliated in their attempts to deal with the hospitals. Research, therefore, must look into all the aspects of these difficult problems.

Service problems

Most services have problems; indeed they are usually described as crises, and the words of Enoch Powell, a former secretary for the Ministry of Health in the UK, are often cited: 'One of the most striking features of the National Health Service is the continual, deafening chorus of complaint which rises day and night from every part of it'.[4] In part, these problems are due to a shortage of resources, and they are made worse by an uncontrolled rise of ambitions and expectations among the professionals. In part, they reflect a more demanding attitude of people in general, and there is a bill to be paid for the past 'exploitation of dedication'. In part, they are due to the increased complexity of a machine which has become too large for human comprehension. In fact, the health service is the largest employer in many countries. The answer usually provided is a rapidly growing administration intended to ensure efficient management, control and equality. Major and unintentional side effects of this are often centralization, bureaucracy, increasing difficulties in political control and public influence at the local level, and decreasing possibilities for innovation and job satisfaction. Obviously, it is extremely difficult to strike a balance between such conflicting goals and interests. This calls for independent and critical research, which may be a nuisance, yet a wise government should support it, because it may help to keep the health service healthy.

Standards and quality of care

Standards are not well defined in medicine, and the professions guard their territories against any attempts to violate clinical autonomy and professional integrity. Research has shown that standards vary enormously, far beyond any reasonable 'normal range', and this is found for most items of service: referral rates, prescriptions, tests, length of stay, etc. This raises two problems: is it possible to define reasonably valid standards, and, if so, is it possible to get them accepted? Both require research.

Prevention

Roughly, one can divide medicine into three parts: prevention, cure and care. What has prevention to offer for the non-infectious diseases? There are perhaps three large problems. The first concerns individuals: How does one make individuals pull their own weight in prevention and brush their teeth, change their life-style, and realize that prevention is not something they get but something they must do?[5] The second concerns the society: how does one improve housing, working conditions and living conditions to make the community a safer, friendlier and healthier place? The third has to do with knowledge, especially epidemiological: what are the preventable causes of cancer, coronary disease and senility? Obviously, much research is needed here.

Public

There are a few more things to say about the public. First, we must teach the public about the potentials and limits of self-care. This requires careful consideration, both medical and educational. Secondly, people will have to rely more on non-professional support from families, friends, neighbours and workmates. This will aid preventive work and becomes essential in the care of the elderly and chronically ill in the community. How does one build and support communities which can and will do this job? Thirdly, we must educate people about attitudes to and expectations from the service. Among other things, this will require a much better and more open complaints procedure and a stronger part for the public in the actual running of the service. It will take research and experimentation to find the way.

This, then, is a list of the more important problems as I see them. The conclusion is obvious to me: none of these problems will go away; they are more likely to grow and multiply. There can be no question, therefore, but that we need health services research to master them.

HOW SHOULD HEALTH SERVICES RESEARCH BE ORGANIZED?

Before I proceed to the next question, a note of caution is in order. Health services research may help to clarify a country's 'national health diseases', but it is no panacea, and we should resist the temptation to oversell it to harassed administrators and politicians.

Goals

Health services research is an instrument for change, a means for improving the service. This is the primary goal, and the research should be planned to achieve this goal. By definition, therefore, health services research should be 'relevant', but it is easy for it to slip off into large projects of little relevance. For research to stay on target, the problem not only must be significant, but it must also have the potential for change within a reasonable time. The time element is important. One should select problems which are likely to come up for consideration, but not so fast that the research is overtaken by political decisions which are already in the making. The secondary goal, of course, is to contribute knowledge of general value.

Problem level

In the great hierarchy of a national health service it is useful to visualize a top political and strategic level and three sub-hierarchies:

   The organization and its managers;

   The clinical operations;

   The technical operations.

One should realize that major political changes in the service are usually not brought about by research. For example, in the UK a laywoman's book— Barbara Robb's *Sans Everything*[6]—probably had greater impact on the care of the elderly than all the research reports. Health services research, possibly with the exclusion of specially commissioned studies of economics and political analysis, is usually aiming for changes in the three sub-hierarchies.

Problem size

It is exciting to work on big problems, but often more comfortable to work on small ones, especially if one has time and money for big research on small problems. In health services research one should look for problems which are important and yet have the potential for change. One should remember that it is probably more healthy for a large organization to improve itself through a continuous series of properly directed small steps, rather than through occasional major upheavals. Karl Popper has this to say about research in general: 'Find out where difficulties arise, and take an interest in disagreements. These are the questions you should take up'.[7]

Research climate

It is obvious from what I have said that research has to steer a difficult course between submissive tail-wagging and unproductive barking and biting. This problem of research climate is usually underestimated, both by research workers and research managers. Research should certainly not direct the service, but it should also not degenerate into a managerial tool.

Inside the service

Changes are usually uncomfortable for a large organization. People feel threatened by them and resist them. Organizations, therefore, tend to become conservative and continue to fight the old battles instead of facing up to the new.[8] A major task for health services research is therefore the study of successful and unsuccessful attempts to change, so that the necessary conditions for successful change can be defined. I believe one condition to be fairly obvious: one must work with the people who are supposed to change, not against them. Put more bluntly: you can reform the service in ten years if you work with the professions, but it will take a hundred years if you work against them. This is a complex issue, because there are of course many vested interests, but I want to make the point that health services research should not be an exercise for epidemiologists and planners. It must be brought inside the service. The research group should work in a service setting, it should choose problems important to the people responsible for the service, and it should involve them—especially the administrators and the doctors—in the work and convince them that it is *their* work. Too often the work is carried out in isolation, reported at special meetings and published in specialist journals, which are read by other research workers but not by the people who must be convinced that the proposed changes are worth while. In many institutions and services the relationship between the clinicians and the administrators is one of 'us against them', and health services research easily ends up as 'their research'. A senior medical citizen told me that he did not know much about health services research, but he 'sure did not like it'. These observations are elementary, but it is amazing to have them confirmed over and over again.

Research has two products, one its results, the other its influence on attitudes and thoughts. In health services research the latter is probably the more important, and its importance will increase if the research is brought inside the service, as 'our' research. Much of it should be carried out by the professions, reported at ordinary meetings and published in general journals. Controlled clinical trials are a good example of a tool which may be used inside the service to promote rational attitudes.[9]

It follows that health services research should choose problems which are important in the local setting. Ideally, the decision-makers and implementers should be involved from the beginning. This will increase their interest and make it more likely that the research eventually will be implemented. The research worker, of course, will work harder if his work is likely to be used. He should remember that his target groups are not his colleagues, but those who can implement his research.

Finally, health services research has an important message to carry outside the service, to make the public and the politicians realize that the health service is fighting 'a battle of priorities,[10] and that research may make this battle more rational.

Old wine in a new bottle?

When I explain the concept of health services research to my colleagues, some get upset because they feel they have done health service research for years, under the label of epidemiology, clinical research or something else. This is a valid point. Health services research is not a new discipline, but rather a new attitude to medicine, medical care and medical research, namely, the attitude that resources are limited and that systematic research must be organized to make the best use of them.

Health services research includes many disciplines, but it is a sterile exercise to construct a general taxonomy for it. Health care consists of people and problems, not of neatly labelled boxes. Yet some sort of system is necessary for those who edit books[11-14] and administer research.[15] In addition, research workers would be pleased to have a map so that they can find their own position and see those of their neighbours. I have studied several schemes with a

TABLE 1

Health services research: types of skills

Medicine (all medical professions)
Epidemiology and statistics
Economics
Social sciences, especially sociology and psychology
Political sciences
Management, manpower and organization studies
Operational research, information systems, computer sciences
Education and behavioural psychology
Technology: buildings, equipment, supplies
Ethics and philosophy

TABLE 2

Health services research: types of problems

Needs and demands
  Surveys, screening
Diseases, disabilities, vulnerable groups
  Surveys, screening, clinical trials
Services
  Primary care, hospital care, outpatient care, long-term and community care
  Utilization of services
  Outcome
  Personnel, technology, costs
Standards and quality of care
  Surveys, clinical trials
Prevention
  Surveys, clinical trials, experiments
Opinions, attitudes and behaviour
  Surveys, attempts to influence
Quality of life
  Surveys, opinions
Self-care, non-professional care and support
  Surveys and experiments

---

mixture of admiration and frustration, and I believe the multidisciplinary activities of health services research cannot be forced into one scheme. At least two schemes are needed, covering types of skills and types of problems (Tables 1, 2). These schemes must be broken down in further detail, and they serve only to suggest what health services research is about. The message clearly is that multidisciplinary research groups must be organized which work inside the service and collaborate with those who do the work of the services.

Teaching

Clearly, it is impossible to set any health service right once and for all. A never-ending series of adjustments will be necessary, and health services research is one of the tools for this job. It must therefore be organized on a permanent basis, and the research group must also teach, so that opinions, attitudes and ambitions can be influenced. The teaching should aim at all professions and levels. It will be more effective if it is based in a medical school.

THE FUTURE

Over the last ten to fifteen years health services research has grown rapidly in the UK and is now getting about 25% of the public money (exclusive of the University Grants Committee money) available for medical research. Major contributions have been made in many fields, for example in epidemiology, clinical trials, the use of hospitals, collaborative research in general practice, and opinions and attitudes (I give no references here, since it would be unfair to mention a few among so many).

Other countries, including Norway, are just facing up to the new situation of limited resources. The first task is to assemble the necessary data bases for assessing the present trends in needs, utilization, costs and manpower. New tasks are obvious, such as:

Measurement of benefits from medical care (outcome studies);
Experiments in prevention;
Standards of quality of medical care;
Quality of life, the human and ethical limitations of medicine;
Expectations, ambitions and spirit of the professions;
Relations between medical and social care;
Long-term studies of vulnerable groups;
Attitudes to self-care and non-professional support in the communities.

The research must be organized on a permanent basis, carried out inside the service, and combined with teaching, preferably as a normal part of the activity of a medical school.

ACKNOWLEDGEMENTS

During the autumn of 1975 I studied health services research in the UK. I thank all the patient people who gave me so much of their time. I also thank the British Council for advice and much help, and the Norwegian Research Council for Science and the Humanities for financial support.

Discussion

Black: What do you mean when you say there is more manpower when money is scarce, Dr Hjort?

Hjort: At the moment, the UK lacks money and has an excess of general manpower. In Norway, we have more money but manpower is severely limited. The health service is affected, because in Norway it uses 20% of the new manpower available every year.

Rogers: This question haunted me throughout my time at the DHSS. In the long run manpower is the most important constraint, and that includes problems arising from distribution of manpower. How do we deal with the problems of the elderly when on our South Coast, for example, one quarter of the population is over sixty-five years of age, and one town even has a third aged over sixty-five. The elderly in those areas may have to have a type of care which is different from a theoretical ideal, and certainly different from the rest of the country. The social services in this country in the last ten years have taken into their employment a substantial proportion of the total increase in available manpower and womanpower. Yet planning for social care by various authorities, including local authorities, suggests a projection of further demand which is totally impossible in terms of the likely available manpower.

Hjort: In Norway, the cost of the social services, including all kinds of social support, is double that of the health services.

Pickering: One of the greatest disasters to hit the health service in the UK was the Salmon Report.[16] This takes our best nurses out of the wards and arms them with pieces of paper which they carry around the corridors until they find a ward sister who is providing coffee, and then they go and interrupt her. The best nurses no longer nurse; they administer. The Committee recognized that their scheme might not work and they recommended that it should be tried out first in a few hospitals. Instead the recommendations were applied wholesale. I always suspected that this must have been due to pressure from the senior nurses.

Hjort: The effects you ascribe to the Salmon Report seem to be happening in all professions. I sometimes visualize the health service as a big army where there is a drift towards the rear lines. These are predictable things, so why should we sit around and let them happen?

Saracci: I see a problem in recruiting people, in particular epidemiologists, with good scientific training and ability for health services research. Many projects in health services research are potentially valuable for the local community concerned but are not of so much general scientific interest, except perhaps for the methodological aspect. At the same time decisions about the community health issues investigated through these projects are taken by administrators and lay representatives of the community (which is as it should be). If this occurs, an epidemiologist who has put aside research of more general interest, such as aetiological studies, to devote himself to research of higher local value, is likely to become frustrated and wish to go back to investigating disease aetiology.

Hjort: I agree that the present system of research easily produces frustration, because the person doing the research work is not responsible for its practical use. Often, valuable work in health services research has no immediate practical use. A good example comes from the comparisons made between health services in different countries: they solve no problems, but they raise important questions, thereby contributing to a more informed and rational climate. I think we must educate ourselves to accept that it is not beneath our status to do this kind of work, and we must organize research in such a way that the potential implementer gets involved. Remember, three things are necessary to make a man change what he is doing: he needs reliable information, he needs time to think about it, and he must not lose face in the operation.

Querido: Medicine is a dynamic system and therefore many facts which one learns in medical school may be less relevant ten years later. I agree that health services research in the curriculum will be very instructive. However to produce a doctor who is able to understand and contribute to change, it seems to me that a change of educational emphasis is needed for medical students. They should participate actively during six months or a year in research, not to make them into research workers but to make them familiar with scientific reasoning.

Professor Arie Querido in Holland was far ahead of his time in research on medical care delivery and I think that was because he was a good physiologist in the first part of his career. He was able to apply the scientific method. The scientific method is becoming increasingly important for general doctors who have to decide for patients whether they are ill or have a disease, or both, and what the causes or effects are or may be. I frequently say that it is much easier to become a heart surgeon than a general practitioner. The general practitioner has to face the problems Dr Eisenberg described earlier (pp. 3-15) whereas the heart surgeon needs more straightforward technical skills. I suppose that we need to have a fresh look at medical education, not only at the curriculum. And of course we have to know where the demands on the health service will fall.

Hjort: I agree that in the long run changes must be made through medical education. On the other hand, I am reluctant to accept that scientific training is necessary for facing up to priorities. After all, consumers have to decide priorities every day, but doctors are excluded from making similar decisions. The problem may often have a fairly simple solution if we are willing to accept the idea that priorities must be assigned.

Marinker: We keep returning to education. If we need education for change we must be concerned with education in scientific method. If research means the application of the scientific method then, in terms of cost–benefit and humanity, we need to teach about it. The difficulty is what to take out of medical education to make room for what you want to put in. There is often a great deal of enthusiasm for putting in something like a year of research for students, but something has first to come out.

Randle: I think that educational change depends on external pressure, and I am curious as to where the pressure is going to come from for this particular change. The development of undergraduate unrest in 1968 or thereabouts led in the UK to dissatisfaction with courses and curricula which could not be ignored. To my view this has been, somewhat surprisingly, of great benefit, because it made teachers focus acutely on what they were doing in their teaching. One of the problems of postgraduate education is that no comparable upheaval has occurred to focus the attention of teachers on what they are doing.

I do not think that health services research will derive much benefit from tinkering with medical education, because I cannot see that doctors will generate the necessary pressure for change. One possibility might be to train health service administrators in universities and allow the pressure to arise from them and their teachers. Pressure should really come from the public but the interposition of the political system between the public and their health service may prevent this. Administration is an area which could apply pressure. I do not like the idea of doctors as sole monitors any more than I like, say, the police as sole monitors of their own work.

Black: Most doctors probably want to be unmonitored, but perhaps monitoring by doctors would be an acceptable compromise.

Hjort: I think that pressure for change must come from doctors themselves. Control has to be either by the profession or by the bureaucracy, so if *we* are not willing to do the job we must accept that the bureaucracy will do it for us.

Fliedner: Our problems in Germany are similar to those you pointed out, Dr Hjort. However, your list of problems (Table 2, p. 159) does not refer to the question of who is doing what, with what type of training and for what purpose. We need to define who is going to be involved in what types and phases of health services because this strongly influences the training of physicians. Their training is still geared largely to curative medicine. We teach medical students very little about ecology, very little about health services and nothing about prevention. There is no glamour in research on preventive medicine, yet it is probably one of the key elements of the future. We also teach students very little about rehabilitation and perhaps Dr Dornhorst's prejudice against physical therapy (p. 90) arises from the general lack of recognition that rehabilitation measures are important. It might be useful to mention an OECD study, *New Directions in Education for Changing Health Care Systems*, which deals systematically with many of the points made here on aspects of educational change.[17]

I want to come back to the question of whether health services research should be within the service or outside, and whether the pressures come from outside or inside. If one of the pressures that has built up over the cost explosion is medical research, those doing medical research should also be responsible for considering the possible social and ethical implications. The German government is developing a programme for 'Research and Technology in the Services of Health' which will be a combined programme of the Ministry of Youth, Family and Health, the Ministry of Science and Technology, and the Ministry of Labour. This will, perhaps, reshuffle our health sciences research efforts. It will have three major thrusts, one of which will be health services research in various areas. I was chairman of the committee advising the government on the intellectual framework for this programme and we thought we should develop a general goal for it first. We asked whether what was wanted was research directed mainly at prolonging life as such (which would perhaps cost more and more money and give less and less benefit). Then we asked what diseases and illnesses impair 'productive' life, that is, life with a fair degree of unimpaired self-fulfilment. One then gets a very different weighting of diseases, as one considers not only their frequency but also the degree of impairment of that 'productive life' they produce. The diseases that head the list in these circumstances are diseases of the respiratory tract, of the vascular system and of the digestive tract, in addition to accidents. In accident research the problem of rehabilitation is of course important. For client-oriented research one should probably consider factors other than morbidity and mortality. Impairment of self-fulfilment and quality of life aspects then become important.

If we want to improve health for the productive life rather than for physical life in terms of years we then come to three sub-priorities which need to be explored. That is, first we should improve present methods and develop new ones for the *prevention, early recognition and diagnosis of disease*, and for *treatment and rehabilitation*. This is probably the most important area for the medical profession but I felt that if we did not plan a place for basic medical research at this stage no money would be committed for it. The second area, the improvement of present methods and the development of new ways of eliminating *environmental influences*, includes the way people behave about their health. This comes back to health maintenance and health education. The third area is devoted to *health care research*.

When productive life is taken as the principal objective, priorities can be set for investment. When we define the disease areas that impair productive life rather than those responsible for most deaths, we get a completely different weighting of research problems. There is room for much basic research, since analysis of the relevant diseases shows that one probably has to provide for three types of research. One type is of long-range importance and would usually affect prevention of disease in our grandchildren. The second type, research directed to diagnosis and treatment, will benefit our children in about ten years from now. The third type, research in rehabilitation and secondary prevention, early recognition and so on, will benefit us within the next five years. All three kinds of research are important, and all three must be supported.

If we look at the relevant disease areas to see which is most important now, in most areas we must conclude that we do not know much about the patho-physiological mechanisms involved. This is the justification for a lot of basic research, but we must realize that the return on that investment will come much later.

Hiatt: Several speakers have referred to the complexity of the problems they discussed. These problems often involve many disciplines. Over the last few decades an extraordinary partnership of biology and medicine has led to great dividends in our understanding of many diseases and our capacity to deal with them. However, many of today's health problems require contributions from a range of other disciplines (as well as the natural sciences), including ethics, economics, decision analysis, statistics and management. Few physicians have been well trained in these spheres, and that will undoubtedly and appropriately continue to be the case, at least for physicians who deal with individual patients. Therefore, a major question that confronts us now, in addition to how medical education should change, is how to interest the most able ethicists, economists, statisticians, etc., in medical and other health-related questions. Dr Hjort suggests that health services research involving experts from other areas ought to be based in medical schools. I agree, but I feel that such an arrangement is incomplete. For example, with notable exceptions, it has not been possible to attract the best biochemists into, say, departments of surgery to do biochemical research in surgery. In general, scholars in a discipline want to have a major foothold in their own disciplinary departments. Further, universities are not set up in such a way as to encourage easy crossing of what are usually rigid departmental lines. Therefore, we must create new institutional arrangements that will permit us to call on the best people from other disciplines to work with us on these problems. I am not, of course, suggesting that managers or economists or statisticians should replace physicians in the approach to crucial problems—we have all been exposed to the silly decisions that can be made in the absence of medical input.

Black: Medical education isn't just a question of producing doctors, of course, but surely we ought to recognize that in the postgraduate sphere they can diverge in many directions. As Dr Hiatt has been saying, we have the same problem with economists, statisticians and so on as we already have with clinical chemists and others who are not medically qualified. The essence of the problem is to recognize equality of status.

Campbell: The German research programme Dr Fliedner has just described (p. 164) is reminiscent of the programme outlined by the Canadian Federal Minister of Health.[18]

Querido: I work on a committee which is trying to define goals for health services research. In The Netherlands at present there is a tendency to confuse research with medical technology and many people are suspicious of medical technology. Therefore there is a tendency to spend the money on health *care* research. Many members of our committee find it difficult to identify the indicators for measuring the quality of health care. It seems to me that research on the health care system can be roughly divided into problems of efficacy and of efficiency. Efficiency has a large component of management and one can study aspects such as whether larger units would be more efficient, whether the teams are properly structured, etc. Efficacy is another matter, but the indicators are indeed very difficult to define. Efficacy depends for a large part on the right decisions being taken by individuals and adequate skills applied. So although health services research is interesting, I don't think that much will come out as far as the quality of care is concerned. It is very much determined through the skills of individuals, and decisions taken by individuals. I mention this as a warning against too high expectations from the results. I prefer to emphasize the educational aspects and to see whether the right mix of knowledge, skills and reasoning is achieved.

Hjort: I agree that it is important not to over-sell health care research. However, the philosophy of limited resources which is built into the concept of health care research is really more important than the results that come from it. This philosophy should penetrate into the service, not to save money, but to give best value for money. This will often lead to better medicine, I believe, because it will emphasize the human aspect of medicine. Therefore, this research should be brought inside medical schools, to give it support and prestige and to facilitate teaching.

References

1. Cooper, M. H. (1975) *Rationing Health Care*, Croom Helm, London
2. Levy, N. B. & Wynbrandt, G. D. (1975) The quality of life on maintenance haemodialysis. *Lancet 1*, 1328-1330
3. Walker, J. H., Thomas, M. & Russell, I. T. (1971) Spina bifida and the parents. *Developmental Medicine and Child Neurology 13*, 462-476
4. Powell, J. E. (1966) *Medicine and Politics*, Pitman Medical, London
5. Illich, I. (1975) *Medical Nemesis*, Calder & Boyars, London
6. Robb, B. (1967) *Sans Everything*, Nelson, London
7. Magee, B. (1973) *Popper*, Fontana/Collins, London
8. Schon, D. A. (1971) *Beyond the Stable State*, Penguin, Harmondsworth, Middlesex
9. Cochrane, A. L. (1972) *Effectiveness and Efficiency: Random Reflections on Health Services*, Nuffield Provincial Hospitals Trust, London
10. Castle, B. (1975) Referred to in *The Times*, October 5
11. McLachlan, G. (ed.) (1971) *Portfolio for Health: The Role and Programme of the DHSS in Health Services Research*, Nuffield Provincial Hospitals Trust/Oxford University Press, London
12. McLachlan, G. (ed.) (1973) *Portfolio for Health 2: The Developing Programme of the DHSS in Health Services Research*, Nuffield Provincial Hospitals Trust/Oxford University Press, London
13. McLachlan, G. (ed.) (1974) *Positions, Movements and Directions in Health Services Research*, Nuffield Provincial Hospitals Trust/Oxford University Press, London
14. Johnson, M. (ed.) (1974) *Medical Sociology in Britain*, British Sociology Association, Medical Sociology Group, Leeds
15. Department of Health and Social Security (1974) *Annual Report on Departmental Research and Development 1974*, HM Stationery Office, London
16. Committee on Senior Nursing Staff Structure (1966) *Report* (Salmon, B. L., chairman), Ministry of Health and Scottish Home & Health Departments / Her Majesty's Stationery Office, London
17. Centre for Educational Research and Innovation (1975) *New Directions in Education for Changing Health Care Systems*, OECD Publications, Paris
18. Lalonde, M. (1974) *A New Perspective on the Health of Canadians*, Govt. of Canada, Ottawa

Client-oriented medicine

Sir DOUGLAS BLACK

Department of Health and Social Security, London

Abstract   Both weak (Illich) and strong (Kerr White, Cochrane) cases have been made for radical changes in medical education and medical practice. The real needs of patients and of the community are considered to be incompletely served by the prevailing emphasis on acute hospital medicine, to the comparative neglect of primary care in the community and of the needs of particular 'client groups', e.g. the mentally and physically handicapped, and the elderly. Inherent in this approach are emphases on information systems related to morbidity rather than to mortality; on 'care' rather than on 'cure'; on quality control relating to 'outcomes' rather than to 'structure' or 'process' of practice; and on controlled trials of both new and accepted forms of treatment.

Difficulties in this approach include the taxonomic incongruity of 'client-group' statistics and the 'disease-system' categories of biomedicine; the therapeutic expectations of the consciously ill; the intellectual interest and the immediacy of specialized clinical practice; and the necessary and profitable links between medical science and the general corpus of science. Nevertheless, and in the full recognition that what is socially desirable may not be scientifically feasible, there is a need in the research context to explore methods of assessing the 'health service priorities' to be attached to biomedical categories. However, these priorities are in themselves multiple, and their relative weighting involves value judgements which are not completely quantifiable.

The title of this paper falls some way short of being self-explanatory, nor is the subject susceptible of summary definition. To an extent, it recognizes the truism (always honourable in the observance, dishonourable in the breach) that the practice of medicine is for the benefit of patients rather than of doctors. This idea could just as well be summarized as 'patient-oriented medicine', but the implication in the title goes beyond this, in recognizing the existence of 'client groups' of patients, whose needs are broadly similar, e.g. the elderly, and the physically and mentally handicapped. Thus extended, the term expresses an attitude that the needs of a community, and of groups within it, for health care may in some way take precedence over the perceived needs of individuals, and *a fortiori* over the professionalism of doctors and others engaged in the provision of care. There is a clear and obvious tension between this attitude and the claims which have been traditionally made for 'clinical freedom', for 'personal medicine', and for 'knowledge for its own sake', irrespective of consequences. This attitude has implications for medical practice, for medical education, and for medical research. It would be foolish to ignore its prevalence and its strength, and the extent to which it has influenced lay opinion. It has been advocated (in my view *ad absurdum*) by Illich,[1] and much more responsibly by Cochrane[2] and Kerr White.[3]

The extreme case, as put forward by Illich,[1] seems to me to fall down sufficiently under the weight of his own advocacy. For example, he says of the decline of tuberculosis, 'chemotherapy played a minor, possibly insignificant, role' (ref. 1, p. 20), and of cardiac catheterization that it 'kills one in fifty people on whom it is performed' (ref. 1, p. 49). His headings include 'Defenceless Patients'; 'Public Control over the Medical Mafia'; 'Trade Union Claims to a Natural Death'; and 'Doctors' Effectiveness—an Illusion'. This is scarcely the language of well-founded and calm debate. Of course, the practice of medicine is neither perfect, nor in the last resort perfectible; but to regard it as an actual conspiracy to deprive mankind of a healthy adjustment to pain, sickness and death is a paranoid transgression of the bounds of common sense. I cannot be alone in failing to accept an argument which concludes 'Increasingly pain-killing turns people into unfeeling spectators of their own decaying selves'.*

Having paid passing tribute to the Mephistopholean role of Illich ('Ich bin der Geist der stets verneint') let us leave the fantasy that accommodation to pain, sickness and death is in some way life-enhancing, and turn to the more sober arguments of Cochrane[2] and Kerr White,[3] who challenge not the validity of professionalized health care but its current effectiveness and efficiency. Magee[5] commends Karl Popper's practice of seeking out the strongest statement of a case which he is about to criticize, and even of fortifying it further, so that it may be 'at its most powerful and appealing'. In humble imitation of this, I shall try to set out the case for a radical reorganization of health care, which would entail among other things a changed emphasis in the aims and

---

* I hope that my reaction to Illich's idea that pain is good for us, and should not be interfered with, has causes deeper than the obvious professional defensiveness. I am encouraged in this hope by a somewhat similar opinion, expressed in a quite different context. Writing of Beethoven's late quartets, Sullivan says: 'To be willing to suffer in order to create is one thing; to realise that one's creation necessitates one's suffering, that suffering is one of the greatest of God's gifts, is almost to reach a mystical solution of the problem of evil, a solution that it is probably for the good of the world that very few people will ever entertain'.[4]

conduct of medical research. I shall rely heavily on paraphrase and quotation, so that as little as possible of the case may be lost.

ARGUMENTS FOR A RE-DIRECTION OF MEDICAL EFFORT

It seems to be a fact of life that new approaches generate new terminologies, so may I clear the ground by explaining the use of some words, common in themselves, but given a special meaning in the context of health care and its assessment. In his Lumleian lecture on 'Monitoring in Medicine', Smart[6] approved the analysis of health care into 'structure', 'process' and 'outcome'. 'Structure' covers the facilities in buildings, equipment, manpower and organization for what is termed the 'delivery of health care'. 'Process' refers to the ways in which these facilities are made use of, and includes 'medical audit', whether this is based on self-assessment, on peer review, or on scrutiny of records. 'Outcome' relates to what is achieved, and, as Smart points out, evaluation of outcome is both crucially important and immensely difficult, because of the need for value judgements on the quality of all outputs short of death. The terms 'effectiveness' and 'efficiency' were introduced as a 'personally invented terminology' by Cochrane,[2] and have gained wide currency. In ordinary usage, they are virtually synonymous, but they have become accepted 'terms of art' with different and fairly precise meanings. Cochrane distinguishes 'two preliminary steps which are essential before the cost–benefit approach becomes a practical possibility'. The first of these is 'to measure the effect of a particular medical action in altering the natural history of a particular disease for the better'. The result of such a measurement indicates the '*effectiveness*' of the action. Summation of the effectiveness of all the courses of action would give the 'effectiveness' of a health service; it would of course be a miracle if the negative sign were totally lacking from this computation. The second step relates to 'the vast problem of the optimum use of personnel and materials in achieving these results. This covers not only problems of treatment, but also those of screening, diagnosis, place of treatment and length of stay, and, if necessary, rehabilitation. To cover all these varied activities I have used the word "*efficiency*".'

This is an important distinction, for me somewhat blurred by the similarity of the terms used. Perhaps I can clarify it for others as well as for myself by suggesting that in essence 'effectiveness' refers to 'outcomes'; 'efficiency' to an amalgam of 'structure' and 'process'.

Kerr White[3] asks the question: 'Why, at this time, are medicine and the provision of health care rapidly becoming a major focus of debate in almost every industrialized society?' In his answer, he instances the dramatic rise in the cost of supporting a health-care establishment; the issues of personal accountability and social responsibility; the 'increasingly evident need to establish priorities for allocating energy and resources in all sectors of the economy'; and the fact that 'there has been little or no improvement in life expectancy for adults since the 1920's. In particular, effective means have not been found for coping with the stubborn complex of chronic and social illnesses that now predominate in the economically advanced countries'. He writes, of course, from the American standpoint; but those factors, with some differences of detail, are generally shared in the developed countries, and are already visible in outline in those which are still developing. Maxwell[7] gives comparative figures which indicate the universality of the 'health care dilemma' in Europe, the USA and the USSR, in spite of varying systems of delivery. Klein[8] considers the sharpening effect of inflation on the resource component of the dilemma, as it affects Britain; and he reveals the inadequacy of the '1% of GNP' index as a measure of health care resources, at a time when the escalation of the 'Growth State' has halted.

The health care dilemma is no doubt many-horned; but if we stick to the conventional pair of horns, and if one of these is the predictable constraint, just mentioned, on the provision of resources, the other clearly concerns the effectiveness and efficiency of their use. To quote Kerr White again, and at some length, for I do not see how the issue could be better put:

'On what basis does a society assign priorities for medicine? Whose values are expressed in the allocation of a nation's energy and resources to improve the quality of life for all its citizens? At the heart of any consideration for medicine's place in contemporary society are the underlying models that give rise to both assumptions and expectations—assumptions on the part of the health-care establishment about the role of science and technology in the provision of health services, and expectations on the part of consumers about what medicine can accomplish and what they must achieve for themselves by modifying their personal behavior.

'Should diseases be likened to ivy growing on the oak tree or are they part of the oak tree itself? Should diseases be regarded as human analogues of defects in an internal-combustion engine or a Swiss watch, or should they be regarded as psychobiological expressions of man evolving within the constraints and potentials contributed from his aliquot of society's gene pool? Are diseases "things" that "happen" to people or are they manifestations of constructive or destructive relations of individuals in their social and physical environment? Depending on our views about the relevance of these contrasting models for understanding health and disease, we modify our behavior, change our expectations, deploy our resources and measure our accomplishments. By resolving these conflicting views we strike a balance in undergraduate medical education between the biological and the social sciences, in graduate medical education between the preparation of technologically based specialists and psychobiologically trained generalists, in medical organization between solo entrepreneurial practice and multispecialist corporate or group practice, and in medical insurance between "catastrophic" coverage of major medical illnesses and "first dollar" coverage of early ambulatory care, anticipatory medicine and counseling'.[3]

Kerr White then goes on to admit 'In the absolute sense there are no right or wrong resolutions of these issues'. He does not, however, in the remainder of his article, conceal his preference for the second model, which gives priority to the expectations of customers, and to the intrinsic, psychobiological concept of 'disease'. Emphasis on the constitutional aspect of disease is no new thing. It can be traced back to the Hippocratic writings; and the interaction aspect crystallized in the apophthegm 'there are no diseases, only sick people' has informed all good clinical practice. But Kerr White and many others see it as newly threatened by 'complex medical technology', and 'super- (or sub-) specialisation', to use the terminology of the critics.

Like Cochrane, Kerr White lays great stress on outcomes. He continues his course of Socratic questioning thus:

'Given the present state of medical science and technology in the context of contemporary industrial communities, what should be the objectives of medical education and medical care? Should medicine adopt the posture that it "fixes" illnesses and "cures" diseases, or should it adopt the posture that it helps people to identify their individual and collective health problems and assists them to resolve or contain them? Should the health-care establishment be judged more on its capacity to investigate and treat abnormal pathology than on its accomplishments in helping patients and their families to understand and manage their problems? What social or even medical utility is to be accorded diagnostic ability if it is not accompanied by effective action and an acceptable outcome? Because we have mastered some procedure, does it follow that society should make it available to all who seek it? To all who can pay for it? To all who need it? Is the new procedure to be preferred over some other form of intervention for the same health problem?'[3]

Having accepted the argument that the costs of intensive hospital treatment are both formidable and rapidly growing, and that many forms of treatment have never been evaluated by controlled trial or indeed on any objective basis stronger than 'clinical opinion', Cochrane and Kerr White both advocate a substantial diversion of resources from the hospital sector to the primary care sector, and from the 'curing' to the 'caring' services. Kerr White sees the need for primary medical care as 'the central problem facing American medicine today'. He does not of course have in mind the old-fashioned general practitioner, working in isolation, and with no access to specialist help. Describing what he wants to see, he says 'This primary-care physician should be well-trained scientifically, particularly in the behavioral sciences. He should know the limits of his capabilities and have access to teams of highly trained sub-specialists supported by ancillary personnel, by technologically sophisticated equipment and particularly by on-line computer regimes that provide timely information about the distribution of clinical manifestations and the efficiency of treatments'.[3] In his concluding chapter on the future of the health service, Cochrane says 'The main change will be the movement of the centre of gravity of medicine from the hospital to the community, associated with a rise in the importance of the GP in relation to the consultant, and the disappearance of the pathologist as the final medical arbiter'.[2] The grounds of this prediction are not clearly stated, but the emphasis on the high cost of hospitals in the earlier chapters suggests that they may be largely financial.

On the 'cure' and 'care' issue, Cochrane is much more explicit, and his arguments are fully set out in his chapter on 'Equality in the health services'.[2] Having made it clear that he is concerned not with quality of treatment but with quality of living, he documents the gross inequality between different types of hospital in staffing and resources. Although Kerr White puts it as a question, he clearly implies that 'resources currently expended on pills, potions and procedures whose benefits or efficacy have never been objectively evaluated' should be 'shifted to the provision of personnel and services to make living with chronic disability more comfortable and dying more dignified'.

Having made a strong egalitarian case for redistribution of the resources, material and human, devoted to health care, both Kerr White and Cochrane recognize that implementation must be based on improved information systems and on widespread evaluation of what is being done and what is proposed to be done. Kerr White lays particular emphasis on information systems, and Cochrane on evaluation by the randomized controlled trial.

Kerr White stresses the inadequacy of conventional mortality statistics as the sole basis of planning. In a particular account of information systems he says 'The question with respect to health services is not how many people are dead, but how many are unable to work, how many are in bed, how many are in pain, how many are not protected against preventable diseases?'[9] It is therefore necessary for conventional vital statistics to be supplemented by hospital activity analysis, by information on sickness benefit, and by analysis of the work-load of general practitioners. Two important tools have already been developed, in the shape of the 'problem-oriented medical record' (Weed[10]) and medical record linkage (Acheson[11]). The Weed record emphasizes the patient's problems, which can seldom be constrained within a single diagnostic label. Medical record linkage protects the integrity of a patient's medical record against the confusions inherent in successive episodes of illness, between which the patient may have changed his doctor, his hospital, and even (increasingly) his home. The development costs of a comprehensive information system are daunting, particularly at present; but planning of services is unrealistic without an adequate information base.

In a penetrating discussion of the nature of evidence, in relation to treatment, Cochrane says 'The oldest, and probably still the commonest form of evidence proffered, is clinical opinion. This varies in value with the ability of the clinician and the width of his experience, but its value must be rated low, because there is no quantitative measurement, no attempt to discover what would have happened if the patients had had no treatment, and every possibility of bias affecting the assessment of the result. It could be described as the simplest (and worst) type of observational evidence'.[2] This low view of unstructured observation leads Cochrane into strong advocacy of the randomized controlled trial (RCT). Although he recognizes the difficulty of eliminating bias, the statistical risks inherent in small numbers and in arbitrary tests of 'significance', and the ethical problems, he nevertheless concludes: 'I believe, however, that the problem of evaluation is the first priority of the NHS and that for this purpose the RCT is much the most satisfactory in spite of its snags. The main job of medical administrators is to make choices between alternatives. To enable them to make the correct choices they must have accurate comparable data about the benefit and cost of the alternatives. These can really only be obtained by an adequately costed RCT'.

The concept of 'client-oriented medicine' has implications for medical education and for medical research. Not surprisingly, Kerr White emphasizes the importance of the behavioural sciences and the statistical approach, and criticizes the preponderance of teaching hospitals, in which 'the focus is largely on acute, episodic illnesses that are usually serious and that can be cured or effectively palliated'. He says further 'The limited exposure of young physicians and their teachers to the full range of ordinary and complex health problems generated by large general populations, and their intense preoccupation with only those patients who are selected to obtain care in teaching hospitals, leave enormous qualitative and quantitative gaps in their experience and inevitably condition their views about the tasks of contemporary medicine'.[3] Any idea that he is alone in these contentions can be dispelled by a glance at the Report of the Royal Commission on Medical Education.[12]

The implications for medical research I shall consider later, but I must now outline some difficulties which I see in the general idea of 'client-oriented medicine'.

SOME CRITICISMS

I hope that I have been scrupulous in presenting the case for client-oriented medicine in its strength, and largely in the words of two of its most influential advocates. I must be equally scrupulous in revealing the biased standpoint from which I view it; I have spent the greater part of my professional life as a hospital consultant—and, worse still—in a teaching hospital. In that capacity, I have had at the very least the strong illusion of dealing with real people and real problems, by no means all of them recondite; so my objectivity may be corrupted by a measure of defensiveness—institutional, I hope, rather than personal.

To look at the broadest issue first, we cannot withhold respect for the egalitarianism and the compassion which are so clearly the emotional springs of the case put forward by Cochrane and Kerr White; and these writers are on firm ground in deploring the personal aggrandisement and the commercialism which can from time to time taint the practice of individual medicine, and which are sometimes given undue prominence by those who purport to 'represent' the profession. But there are other values in medicine which cannot be neglected —the pursuit of excellence in practice, the desire to add to knowledge, the satisfaction of direct contact with people rather than with groups. These have been powerful factors in determining the way in which medicine has developed, and they must be taken into account in assessing the practicality of changing direction in the way proposed. Alan Williams has put the essence of the difficulty rather well:

'In the medical field two distinct kinds of choice arise: one at the clinical level and the other in the planning process. At the point of contact with a particular patient, a doctor's duty is to do the best he can for that patient within the confines of existing knowledge and facilities. In the planning process, on the other hand, the concern is with large groups of potential patients at some future date, and with decisions that will to some extent determine what the confines of existing knowledge and facilities will be at that date'.[13]

From a considerable experience of medical students, and of candidates for entry to medical school, I have little doubt that the great majority see medicine in terms of clinical practice. In spite of considerable exposure to the biomedical sciences, only a minority of students are even prepared to test their aptitude for medical research, let alone make a career of it. By the same token, while I agree with the need for greater exposure of students, at an early stage of the curriculum, to the behavioural and statistical disciplines basic to community medicine, the effectiveness of this in determining their ultimate choice of career seems to me doubtful. The recognition of community medicine as a specialty, and the establishment of an adequate career structure, have of course removed two important barriers to recruitment; and in this country the Faculty of Community Medicine affords a home for the new specialty. A heavy responsibility rests on the Departments of Social and Preventive Medicine in the medical schools to provide the stimulus and leadership needed to encourage students, including some of the best, to take advantage of these new opportunities. In my judgement, however, it will be some years before adequate numbers of students are sufficiently excited by the challenges and opportunities of community medicine to make this a priority choice of career; and this has clear implications for the time-span over which the patterns of health care can be radically altered.

Problems of recruitment to community medicine aside, implementation of the proposals inherent in 'client-oriented medicine' would have implications for clinical practice which might arouse professional resistance. Cochrane (ref. 2, pp. 81–83) faces this issue frankly. He sees that as a result of objective trials, the indications for prescription, diagnostic tests, and admission to and length of stay in hospital, will become more clearly defined—'a sort of "par for the course" associated with each group of signs and symptoms will be established, and those doctors with too many "strokes" above or below "par" will be asked to justify themselves before their peers'. He also advocates financial restriction on the introduction of costly facilities which have not been evaluated in terms of their outcome. These recommendations seem to me personally to be just and fair; but his lines will not be easily held against the professional defenders of 'freedom of clinical practice', and the activities of powerful pressure groups who may equate the latest and/or the most expensive with the best.

Although Kerr White[3] instances the lack of improvement in life expectancy as one of the causes of dissatisfaction with health care, Cochrane (ref. 2, p. 14) lessens the security of this base by saying of his table giving the time course of life expectancy 'This gives a gloomy picture indeed, particularly for males, but it is of course a very unfair one. The NHS cannot be blamed if there has been an increased incidence of a disease for which there is no effective means of prevention or treatment, although, of course, it could be criticised if it were using ineffective preventive or therapeutic measures in such cases'. Another advocate of a more planned approach to health care (Fuchs), writing from an economic standpoint, spells out more clearly the limitations of what can be expected from the client-oriented approach:

'Implementation of these recommendations should have a significant impact on the problems of *cost and access*. They should not be expected, however, to produce a dramatic improvement in the overall *health* of the population. Such improvement will more likely come as a result of advances in medical knowledge or of changes in human behavior. By changing institutions and creating new programs we can make medical care more accessible and deliver it more efficiently, but the greatest potential in improving health lies in what we do and don't do for and to ourselves. The choice is ours'.[14]

Present-day practice in Britain does not fully bear out the sharpness of the distinctions made between 'cure' and 'care', and between primary and hospital care. A good deal of the practice in district hospitals could be classified as 'care' rather than 'cure'; and the teaching hospitals in general have a considerable component of 'emergency admissions', and a general outpatient practice, which blurs their image as 'over-specialized institutions'. In the smaller centres in this country, there are good working relationships between the family doctor and the hospital specialist, who may undertake domiciliary visits and visits to health centres; while in the large conurbations, a substantial part of the burden of emergency primary care falls on the casualty departments of the hospitals.

Finally, it seems reasonable in considering client-oriented medicine to take some account of the expectations of patients. Fuchs[14] introduces one of his chapters with a dramatic quotation: 'The hospital has evolved from a House of Despair avoided by all but the impoverished sick to a House of Hope to which all roads lead in time of crisis—be it somatic, psychic or social in origin'. While improvements in primary care should lessen this attitude, there is little doubt that the expectations of many patients are centred on a prompt referral to a well-equipped hospital.

Moreover, patients in developed countries expect to be seen by doctors (of the shod variety) and not, or not exclusively, by the class of aides known in America as 'physician-extenders'. Whereas actual experience[15] showed that diagnostic accuracy can be sensibly improved by 'the acquisition of detailed and predefined data' by a non-medically qualified assistant, most patients in the same study would not have been willing to forgo the subsequent interview with a doctor. The assistant in this study had undergone 'an intensive training period of around three months'—there may be an element of incongruity in general proposals which combine an advocacy of 'physician-extenders' with a mistrust of 'over-specialization'. Perhaps the expectations of patients are in this respect soundly based, that they wish the programmed interview by a specialized assistant to be 'covered' by a generally-trained doctor.

IMPLICATIONS FOR RESEARCH

In drawing attention to some of the difficulties in the implementation of 'client-oriented medicine', I have not sought to undermine the positive elements of the case that more attention should be paid to the provision of care so that the most effective use can be made of limited resources. On this basis, I would fully endorse the plea made by Cochrane[2] for an expansion of applied research devoted to this end; if goodwill is to be translated into good practice, the process must be controlled by sound information on what is needed, and by the evaluation of innovations in care, before they are generalized. The problems encountered in this type of research are different from those of biomedical research; the approach to them involves other disciplines—those of epidemiology, economics, operational research, and the social sciences. They are not, however, lacking in interest or in difficulty, and the objectivity of workers on these problems is subject to strains which do not commonly affect the biomedical worker. The formulation of the questions to be answered may be the most difficult part of the whole task.

Having I hope left no doubt of my commitment to the encouragement of health services research, I must rebut, as strongly as I can, two suggestions which are sometimes made.

The first of these is that resources and people should somehow be 'diverted' from biomedical research to health services research. My main objection to this relates to people—while both forms of research are labour-intensive, health services research perhaps rather more so, the training and skills involved are distinctly different, and redeployment over such a wide gap of disciplines is simply not practical. Resource pressures could of course have a long-term effect, by influencing career prospects; but to strengthen health services research *at the expense of biomedical research* would be, in my view, counter-productive to the quality of care, as we would be delaying further discoveries of the kind so well documented by Perutz,[16] which have transformed what can be done for actual patients.

The second, more limited, suggestion is that 'health service priorities' should determine the directions in which biomedical research should be prosecuted. There is a commonsense flavour about this which makes it attractive at a high level of generality. It is usually, and on the whole effectively, combatted by drawing attention to the constraints imposed by scientific feasibility—the 'state of the art'—and the presence or absence of suitable workers. But there is a further difficulty—that of defining 'health service priorities'. Here, the client-group approach, important as it is in service provision, is not particularly helpful, because of the way in which biomedical categories cut across client groups. To give obvious examples, bronchitis can affect all client groups; and on the other hand the ills of the elderly can rarely be constrained within any single biomedical category. An alternative approach is to look at various indices of the burden imposed on the health services by a range of biomedical categories.[17] The main difficulty in this approach is that the different indices produce widely differing rank orders of biomedical categories. For simplicity, I shall illustrate this by giving only the top-ranking cause for each of the five indices which we have used:

Index	Biomedical category	% of total burden
Inpatient days	Mental illness	31.3
Outpatient referrals	Neurological disorders	9.8
General practitioner consultations	Respiratory infections	16.0
Sickness-benefit days	Bronchitis and asthma	11.5
Loss of life expectancy	Ischaemic heart disease	21.5

It is, of course, possible to cost these indices, and by the exercise of economic rigour to evade the value judgements of comparing primary care, hospital usage, loss of earnings, 'misery', and mortality. But would this be a generally acceptable approach? And would it be better than accepting the estimates of wise clinicians on the relative importance of diseases? My answer to the second of these questions is 'Yes'; but to the first of them 'Don't know'.

CONCLUSION

I remember some years ago starting a book by saying 'Medicine means different things to a doctor, to a patient, and to a lay person who is not ill'.[18] More recently, Dingle[19] has expressed a similar idea: 'The most prevalent diseases are not the well-known causes of death. Precisely what they are depends to a surprising degree on whether they are perceived by patients, by physicians or by vital statisticians'. I think I would now recognize that the implied unity of outlook in the medical profession was a gross over-simplification. There have always been doctors who have viewed medicine in a wider social context; but in the past decade this viewpoint has become better organized, more clearly expressed, and correspondingly more influential. It is perhaps more apparent that 'advances in medicine' are not all of one kind. Without ceasing in any way to regard clinical care as the central preoccupation of the doctor, I personally welcome the movement to bring the assessment of outcomes, in the broadest sense of the word, within the ambit of objective scientific scrutiny.

Discussion

Bull: If the client is the general public, and we are talking in the UK of the expenditure of public money, then the client is being placed in the situation of the politician. Political pressures tend to give rise to demands for research in which no account is taken of the basic knowledge which would enable a particular problem to be solved. It leads to such nonsense as 1 % of GNP being demanded for cancer research. That sort of pressure must be avoided by some buffer system. At the moment the buffer system in the UK is the Department of Health and Social Security. But the DHSS is very near the political pressure front and I don't think it is capable of resisting severe pressures from un-informed pressure groups on such things as cancer, deafness and so on. This has to be dealt with in deciding the method of control of client-oriented research. If the client were simply the DHSS, client-oriented research would be abso-lutely splendid, but how do you resist the pressures which lead to demands which are not realistic?

Black: One needs first a system with an element of stability in it; without that one is completely defenceless. The efforts at quantitation of burdens which I described are something in the nature of a defensive mechanism. We need to be able to show pressure groups the true proportion of suffering caused by the problem that interests them, in relation to total suffering. The most important thing, as you indicate, is that recognizing a need still leaves us a long way from being able to do anything about it. My own belief is that priorities, if one can assess them, ought to be one component of the mix. Any progress towards a valid delineation of social priorities would probably help.

Dickinson: Maybe we should not write off the public entirely. Dr Randle said earlier (p. 163) that either the administrative structures of the health service or clinicians themselves should keep taking long hard looks at what is happen-ing. One of the few good features emerging from the reorganization of the health services in the UK is that in a district of perhaps 150000 people it is possible for everyone working in the health services there to know everybody else. Furthermore, consumer groups (the Community Health Councils) are associated with the districts as scrutineers of the health services and of the way resources are distributed between primary health care, general hospitals, research geriatric hospitals, mental hospitals and so on. They have investigative powers and some delaying powers. Although many Councils are still finding their feet, some have already begun to make substantial contributions, as lay people, to helping doctors with difficult problems. The treatment of one patient with haemophilia during one weekend recently at a hospital in London cost about £ 9000 in drugs. The hospital then had to stop supplying drugs for out-patients for three months to recoup and balance its budget. This caused much inconvenience to and waste of time by its patients. Another example is that so many pacemakers were being inserted at one hospital that the district administrator said that the case for this would have to be argued out before further pacemakers could be bought. This sort of thing faces doctors with the most intolerable problems, and our lay colleagues might help us to take a slightly less emotional view. We should see Community Health Councils and similar organizations as allies of the medical profession, and encourage and use them as much as possible.

Campbell: In Ontario we have been trying to involve other people in such decisions and we are also trying to decentralize those decisions, bringing them into the community. It is hard work but very rewarding when the community helps with these matters.

I hope that somebody will make a positive and competent statement about cost. This meeting is about research and practice and there has been a bit of internecine warfare about whose research is most cost-effective. I am confident that all forms of biomedical research are an extremely 'good buy' if the results of research are properly harnessed to health care.

Woodruff: If someone puts to sea in a rowing boat when force 9 gales are predicted, or climbs a mountain when blizzards are forecast, nobody seems to question the cost of mounting a rescue operation. We must look at haemophilia and so on in the context of the other expensive exercises which may save just one person.

References

[1] ILLICH, I. (1975) *Medical Nemesis*, Calder & Boyars, London
[2] COCHRANE, A. L. (1972)   *Effectiveness and Efficiency: Random Reflections on Health Services*, Nuffield Provincial Hospitals Trust/Oxford University Press, London
[3] WHITE, K. L. (1973) Life and death and medicine. *Scientific American 229*, 22-33
[4] SULLIVAN, J. W. N. (1964) *Beethoven: his Spiritual Development*, Unwin, London (first published by Cape, 1927).
[5] MAGEE, B. (1973) *Popper*, Fontana/Collins, London
[6] SMART, G. A. (1975) Monitoring in medicine. *Journal of the Royal College of Physicians of London 9*, 355-370
[7] MAXWELL, R. (1976) *Health Care—the Growing Dilemma* (McKinsey Survey Report), 2nd edn., McKinsey, New York
[8] KLEIN, R. (1975) The national health service, in *Inflation and Priorities* (Klein, R., ed.), pp. 83-104. Centre for Studies in Social Policy, London
[9] WHITE, K. L. (1972) Epidemiologic intelligence requirements for planning personal health services. *Acta Socio-medica Scandinavica 2-3*, 143-151
[10] WEED, L. L. (1968) Medical records that guide and teach. *New England Journal of Medicine 278*, 593-600; 652-657
[11] ACHESON, E. D. (1967) *Medical Record Linkage*, Nuffield Provincial Hospitals Trust/ Oxford University Press, London

12 TODD, A. R. (1968) *Report of the Royal Commission on Medical Education*, HM Stationery Office, London
13 WILLIAMS, A. (1974) The cost-benefit approach. *British Medical Bulletin 30*, 252-256
14 FUCHS, V. R. (1974) *Who Shall Live? Health, Economics and Social Choice*, Basic Books, New York
15 HORROCKS, J. C. & DE DOMBAL, F. T. (1975) Diagnosis of dyspepsia from data collected by a physican's assistant. *British Medical Journal 3*, 421-423
16 PERUTZ, M. F. (1972) Health and the Medical Research Council. *Nature (London) 235*, 191-192
17 BLACK, D. A. K. & POLE, J. D. (1975) Priorities in biomedical research: indices of burden. *British Journal of Preventive and Social Medicine 23*, 222-227
18 BLACK, D. A. K. (1968) *The Logic of Medicine*, Oliver and Boyd, Edinburgh
19 DINGLE, J. H. (1973) The ills of man. *Scientific American 223*, 77-84

Government needs and public expectations

Sir PHILIP ROGERS

(Formerly at) Department of Health and Social Security, London

Abstract The priorities for research which emerge from looking at the health needs of patients collectively are examined here. Priorities, however imperfect, are discernible when the five indices of where the main burdens on the health services lie are examined; those indices are inpatient days, outpatient referrals, general practitioner consultations, sickness-benefit days, and loss of life expectancy. Housing, employment, nutrition, etc., are equally relevant to health and to the question of priorities in medical research. It is important in dealing with government needs and public expectations to be clear what health and social services cannot do and what people must do for themselves.

When Dr Wolstenholme was inviting people to this symposium he suggested briefly what it might cover. His key opening sentence was 'It seems to me desirable to begin with the patient'. Clearly that is right; and indeed I go on from there to suggest that we must also end with the patient. For the most part others here have, necessarily and rightly, started with the particular problems of the research itself. Now that the symposium is nearing its close I would like, from a different viewpoint, to go further and consider whether, to quote again from Dr Wolstenholme's letter, 'we derive for clinical practice all we might from the whole wealth of research'. This seems to be in full accord with my suggestion that we end with the patient: in other words, the end—the object both of the research and of clinical practice—is the health of the individual patient or groups of patients.

In this end is my beginning. My task, as the title of my paper shows, is to look at this problem not from the point of view of the research worker but, starting with the patients collectively, to see what light, what guidance, can be obtained from that examination to help research workers in approaching their task of 'beginning with the patient'. What then are the government and public needs in research and how, on the one hand, can the research which is carried

185

out be related to those needs and how, on the other hand, can the public be better informed in regard to the nature, time-scale and costs of that research —costs in money and, most important of all, in rare skilled manpower? It is necessary first to dispel any idea that the 'Government' about whose needs I speak is for this particular purpose a homogeneous whole. The needs of its separate parts, even in the field of medical research alone, are disparate. It is obvious enough that from the point of view of the Ministry of Health one would wish work in biomedical research to correspond, where practicable, to the relative burdens on the health services of various groups, for example, the aged, the mentally and physically handicapped, the chronically ill and so on. But the needs of, say, the Ministry of Agriculture for medical research on the effect of food additives, or the Department of Energy for research on the lead content of petrol, or the Department of Industry for research on the health hazards of the manufacture of, say, polyvinylchloride may—and indeed do—differ largely from such priorities as might derive from looking at the extent of particular illnesses, the suffering of individual patients, and the burden on the National Health Service. Yet these are all equally legitimate needs of the government in the light of the broad interests of the nation. Within any one or indeed all of these fields there is moreover a dichotomy between the political needs of the government of the day and the longer-term needs deriving from the time-scales of research and of service provision, both for the most part substantially longer than the life-time of any one and often of any two or three governments. But since government, especially in a democracy but ultimately everywhere, rests upon consent, Government must be responsive to public pressure and those of us who think of our work in government solely in the longer-term ignore that at our peril.

It is here that it is of particular importance to achieve better public under-standing of the possibilities and the time-scale and the costs of research. I would hope that such understanding would also minimize, if not entirely avoid, those sudden public and therefore governmental panics which from time to time have distorted what most of us here today would probably regard as rational priorities in research. I hope it is not unfair comment to suggest that there have been occasions when the early publication of initial hypotheses deriving from incomplete research have contributed to those panics. Even if the final impact on the public comes from journalists rather than from science, it is the scientist who has, as it were, kindled the fire by a 'preliminary communication'—and perhaps added fuel to it later by multiple publication. It is not always possible to distinguish rigidly between laudable dissemination of results and less creditable indulgence in the race for priority.

However all these paragovernmental aspects range so widely that it may be most helpful if at this symposium I concentrate on the long-term needs of a Ministry of Health (a name which I use deliberately to narrow the scope, despite our proper title of Department of Health and Social Security) as a basis on which these aspects can be determined, and on the need for common ground between the desire of government to see research effort oriented towards socially and economically desirable objectives on the one hand and the need for the 'freedom' of medical research on the other.

What does a health department need for research? Let me seek to deal with that first in specifically medical terms. I propose to range more widely thereafter in considering other aspects of social provision which I suggest are equally important to health.

First, factual information (as opposed to value judgements) is needed on where the major burdens lie. Basically this is a question of information systems and the epidemiological approach. Our Chairman, Sir Douglas Black, has already done some work in this field,[1] and I hope he will forgive me if I shamelessly draw on work that he and one of our economist colleagues have done. In considering the burden of categories of illness, one can use indices related to the use of resources from the statistics on inpatient days, outpatient referrals and general practitioner consultations. For morbidity the sickness benefit days offer a useful though far from infallible guide, and for mortality, loss of life expectancy is the obvious index. One can then take, for each of these five indices, the burden imposed by each of the categories of disease according to the international classification, using them both in absolute terms and as a percentage of the total burden from that cause. It is not necessary for me to spell out the uncertainties of such an approach, particularly those arising from the uncertainty of diagnosis and from the further major problem of the use of services for preventive and screening procedures. There are, furthermore, significantly different results from each of the five indices used. Yet, when all this is taken into account, it is surely significant and highly relevant to my thesis that in each case more than half the burden on health resources is accounted for by comparatively few categories of disease. This is seen at its most extreme in hospital bed occupancy, about half of which is accounted for by mental illness and mental handicap alone. This of course gives a misleading picture of total patient needs—though it is relevant in considering the burden on NHS resources and therefore the extent to which the needs of other patients can or cannot be met from available resources. Even in the category of bed occupancy, moreover, there is a bias in that 'short stay' conditions (such as attempted suicide or major emergency operations) impose a more intensive burden on assessment and care than does chronic illness. But even if we take the most diverse group, that of consultations with general practitioners, it is surely significant in considering priorities that half the burden is accounted for by only nine categories of disease and that only fifteen categories each account for 2% or more of the total burden.

Apart from the inherent imperfections of the data it will of course be clear that only broad indications of priority could in any event be drawn from such material. For example, different types of burden have been evaluated—emphasis on the hospital burden alone would be different on the two different criteria of bed occupancy and outpatient work, and the burden on primary care is different again. Moreover the indices based on the use of resources would suggest priorities different from those based on 'need', as reflected in morbidity and mortality. The possibility and the propriety of making a value judgement between resource saving, the avoidance of suffering, and the prolongation of life are both open to question. A further point of substance is that there are conditions which cause much suffering but which account for only a small part of resource usage, morbidity and mortality. For example the highest percentage of any indices of burden accounted for by eye diseases is only 1.28% (general practice consultations); ear diseases, including deafness, reach their highest percentage of only 2.60 of the same index. Yet these are conditions of undeniable importance. Moreover, the data inevitably reflect what is being done with existing resources and what is happening to people. We cannot assume that 'whatever is, is right'. Lastly, there is the point with which all here will be extremely familiar, that is that a clear service need for research cannot be equated with the likelihood of that research being profitable.

Mental handicap is very much a case in point. The problems involved may be insoluble in present circumstances, there may be a lack of skilled workers, there may be stultification of research by either a lack or a superfluity of suitable patients—and so on.

Yet, when all these qualifications are made, I suggest that they do not form an excuse for abandoning the attempt to define priorities for biomedical research derived from service needs. I would regard such an approach as anarchy or despair.

I turn now from the factual information to the problem of 'early warning' of advances which will carry resource implications. When for example hospital provision has to be planned on a ten to twenty-year basis this can be of crucial importance though also a matter of extreme difficulty and uncertainty. One cannot assume that all the future equivalents of the tuberculosis sanatoria of yester-year can necessarily be put to good use—yet they may absorb very large resources meanwhile.

Clearly we need to evaluate service provision, through health services research. What are the best means of delivering health care? 'Best' must include both the most effective and the relatively most sparing of resources, that is, the most cost-effective.

We need factual information on models of service provision, through operational research. This is a difficult field and I do not myself believe that in major matters it can go further than suggesting the implications of various models of health provision. Yet those suggestions may be of the utmost importance and can all too easily fail to be recognized if we do not employ this weapon in our armoury. It is, for example, an approach which we in the DHSS found most valuable in our study of the need for community hospitals in relation to District General Hospitals.

This said, it is one thing to have all this information on which to base a reasoned approach to priorities. It is quite another to identify and formulate research projects related to those choices of priority and of policy. Furthermore, when much of our planning of service provision is done on the basis of client groups, their needs are bound to contrast sharply with the disease-oriented nature of biomedical research. It is in these last two aspects that we must seek the common ground to which I referred earlier, between the freedom of medical research on the one hand and its orientation towards 'socially desirable objectives' on the other. This is only possible through the continuing dialogue between those concerned on each side, founded on the mutual respect of each side for the views and the importance of the other.

I shall turn now from this short disquisition on government needs in the field of medical research to those wider social issues which, as I suggested earlier, may be of equal or even greater importance to health, and to the relationship of these to public expectation. It has long been a commonplace that during the last hundred years the health of the population has owed more to the sewage engineer and to the growth of wealth which permits better nutrition than to the efforts of those of us concerned with medical care. I do not propose to dwell on that: but I would like to draw your attention to the problems which are particularly acute as seen from the seat I recently occupied at the Department of Health and Social Security—problems on the relationship of housing, employment and education to health in its widest sense.

In terms of priority and the use of resources for promoting health, there are areas and times when more might be achieved by housing than by hospitals, particularly for such groups as the elderly or the physically handicapped. Employment may be of the greatest importance to health, not only in the obvious field of income and the consequential supply of food, clothing and shelter, but also in relation to mental health. In particular, what about the employment of the elderly, and have we in our social provision neglected this sphere in considering even their physical health? Nor, in referring to education, do I have in mind the relatively narrow if important field of social adjustment which is relevant to the wider health of the community. To take the other side of the coin, what has been the effect on education, and indeed more widely, of a much-vaunted and indeed rightly valued improvement in the feeding of children which led to earlier and better physical growth? Has this led to earlier physical maturity and has this exacerbated the problems of mental and emotional adjustment in early adolescence? Has this had any influence on social *mores* and permissiveness? Have these in turn had any influence on sexually transmitted diseases, the extent of abortion among young girls, or the growing consumption of alcohol by the young? Please do not misunderstand me. I am not even suggesting a necessary causal relationship, let alone suggesting that such factors are major determinants of disease or illness. But these are fields where prejudices masquerade as value judgements and the short answer is surely that in fact we do not know. To take the issue more widely still, how far are questions of what one might broadly term social anthropology relevant to health even in a narrow sense—for example, the effect on communities of uprooting them from slums and rehousing them in entire blocks, whether these be tower or garden city, and the effect of the post-war explosion in the employment of married women on the care of children, to name only two fields—?

You may reasonably comment at this point that all this may be quite true but what has it got to do with the theme of this symposium on research and medical practice? I suggest that medical research has in fact a substantial part to play even in these fields as well as in relation to the problem of specific diseases. Take the social problem of child abuse and child battering. This is not only an issue for doctors in having to identify the cases and cooperate with other professions in dealing with the problem when found. There is a field for research before the abuse takes place. Study of intensive therapeutic work with families in which child abuse had occurred has suggested that bonding failure is related in part to the pregnancy, perinatal experience, and early ill-health of the abused child and parents.[2] Thus the treatment of parents during pregnancy, the perinatal period and early infancy may well be fruitful in the prevention of child abuse. There are surely many fields within the area of the broad social problems to which I have referred where medical research is at the least an essential component of any broad attack on the problem.

As my last topic I return to the problem of public expectations. I have referred already to the dangers, inherent in the crisis approach, that arise from publicized fear; that approach is all too often taken by the media, or through narrowly based pressure groups. There is a need for a system, with some inherent stability though not of course immobility, for the determination of priorities in research. There is the complex relationship between need, demand

and provision. Provision may always be less than demand, but is either (or both) necessarily less than need, as is commonly supposed? A very distorted view of priorities could be obtained if we looked at the patient as a mere passive recipient of health care, for a considerable part at least of ill-health today is self-induced, e.g. smoking, lack of care in driving, sexually transmitted diseases, or even obesity. No perfect equation of need, demand and provision is ever likely to be attainable, even apart from constraints on manpower and resources. At this point, the name Illich also springs to mind. So far no Illich has yet written, as far as I am aware, about social as opposed to health provision, yet his approach may not be without relevance there too—and relevant directly to health, both physical and mental.

I have sought to touch on a range of problems in health, taken in its widest sense, as seen from the problem of someone in government in a central position dealing with health and the related social services. I have referred to the uncertainties which will always be with us about the paths we should take. Yet, at the end of each day, someone has to decide what resources must be provided, and how they should be provided and where, whether those resources be in research or in other fields. I hope that you will agree with me that it is better constantly to search for a rational system of priorities for determining the use of resources, imperfect though those priorities must necessarily be, than to let those resources be frittered away meeting needs or demands that present them- selves haphazardly. I regard it as equally important, in dealing with govern- ment needs and public expectations, to be less chicken-hearted than we are at present in saying what the health and social services cannot do and what people must do for themselves.

Discussion

Black: If, for want of any other sensible way, one gives equal weight to the several burdens imposed by the fifty-three commonest kinds of illness, one finds that only about fifteen of them account for two-thirds of the total burden.[1] Of course one could, by choosing narrower or broader categories of illness, readily expand that number to twenty or reduce it to twelve—the selection is important.

My background in electrolyte and renal physiology is perhaps not ideal when it comes to dealing with social problems, but I am totally convinced that these are important. The great difficulty is getting people to tackle them objectively. Much of what is said amounts to little more than political and sociological asseveration. There are signs that critiques of sociological investigation are improving, and this is to be welcomed.

Eisenberg: It seems essential for national health services to consider those social factors that determine health-care-seeking behaviour: that is, what makes the patient decide to come to doctors or other health service personnel. In housing projects where young married couples live with children and almost no elderly relatives, there is no advice to be had when a first child becomes ill. Inexperienced mothers cannot tell the difference between very ill and mildly ill children so they turn to health personnel. If we propose that the family should assume burdens which are now inappropriately displaced onto the health system, we need to understand the nature of the contemporary family. In the US one in every 2.3 marriages ends in divorce; 56% of married women are in the labour force; 30% of children under six years have working mothers. The family with a female head is almost always at a severe economic disadvantage. Advice to mothers about playing with their children assumes that they are at home to play with them. These issues are political and involve questions of values and priorities. Our present government in the US considers that one way of winning the war against inflation is to tolerate a high unemployment rate. I believe that there ought to be some more equitable distribution of the burden, but that is my political conviction, not the President's.

In a study by Roghmann and Haggerty,[3] mothers kept diaries of stressful events; analysis revealed that mothers sought medical advice for a child (but not for themselves) more often if there had been a stressful event in the family that day. The child's illness was not necessarily produced by the stress but at the least the mother's behaviour correlated with stress. Thus, in addition to causal research, one needs to look at social patterns of health and at what other remedies are available within communities in order to restore what the extended family once supplied.

In the US one in five families moves every year; on average, no one stays in the same house for more than five years. The nuclear family obviously becomes the prototypical family and relatives are not available. Can we reinvent grandmothers? Grandmothers used to be an enormously important part of the socialization process. In one American town recently, a newly arrived family advertised in the newspaper for a set of foster grandparents who might be available on a friendly basis. Shouldn't housing be planned so that a certain number of the elderly live where the young are? We should think of ways of making it easier for people to get together, though not everything responds to planning. We must look at the social group and all the other health-seeking and health-providing behaviours that come before as well as after the medical enterprise or we may fail to respond to public needs. Those needs are constantly being displaced onto a system that is not now appropriate for them.

Rogers: I wholly agree about the nuclear family. It is a paradox that on the one hand the present conventional family is so small, while on the other the number of elderly people who lack an occupation which is relevant to their happiness and health is growing. These two factors should certainly be kept in mind, particularly in housing planning.

Dornhorst: The influence of social factors on health is now more widely recognized in the medical profession but I doubt whether it is the doctor's job to pursue the necessary research. He should be aware of the problems and take an interest in the answers, but it is really the field of medical sociologists. Unfortunately, within sociology, the status of medical sociology is low; it is considered too applied and not intellectual enough, with people producing useful data instead of a large conceptual model. Indeed the MRC Unit of Sociology has difficulty in recruitment for this reason. I think it is a mistake to try and train doctors as medical sociologists. It is wasteful to put the medical man to work on questions about which he lacks the appropriate disciplinary training, and to do both types of work is also wasteful.

Black: I agree with that. Sociology is a very young science compared with medicine and I hope that sociologists will soon decide to concentrate on society as it exists, as something that can be improved piecemeal rather than made the subject of an experiment in radical total change, beginning with destruction even of the things that work reasonably well.

Rogers: I agree that doctors should be interested in these problems. I did not mean to suggest that they should turn themselves into sociologists.

Randle: Recent trends towards integrated curricula for medical education have tended to isolate medical students from other groups in non-collegiate universities, as mentioned earlier (p. 70). I would doubt whether this is entirely desirable. The contacts undergraduates make with other groups of students are more lasting and rather different from contacts made later in life. People's minds at that age are more receptive and more flexible than later. Medical students should be thrown into contact with other groups of students whose work may then be seen to be relevant to the problems of medicine.

Earlier (p. 163) I said that in the UK we should try to train health service administrators in places where they would come into contact with medical students and others with relevant special interests. Administration is sometimes bad because it is intellectually deprived, and perhaps bureaucracy is administration without research. It seems to me important that administrators should have research activities of their own. I find it is much easier to deal with administrators who have knowledge deriving from their own research on a problem than with administrators who are entirely dependent on other people for ideas.

Rogers: I agree, but there are varied views on how to train administrators.

I think they should have a broad education, with training afterwards, and it is at this stage that they could mix with doctors. This is what the DHSS is trying to do.

Woodruff: One reason why many people go on smoking cigarettes, for example, is that they think they themselves will escape the harmful results—other people may get lung cancer, not them. Medicine should analyse the reasons for this, which in a way is pathological behaviour. Another reason why self-help is diminishing is perhaps because, particularly in the UK, we tend to look to the state to provide all our welfare needs. To a certain extent irresponsibility and lack of self-help involve an element of mental disorder. No doctor, not even a surgeon, can fail to be interested in these problems, even though he is not a sociologist; indeed we have a responsibility to be interested in them.

Saracci: Self-help is rightly going to become more and more important, in different forms within different frameworks or different societies. But we should not fall into the mistake of using self-help as an easy way to push all the responsibility onto individuals. In cigarette smoking, for example, we can hardly expect people to help themselves when the incentives are all wrong. The effort should be in the direction of identifying and developing social conditions in which people become able to exercise self-help. In the occupational setting one cannot ask the worker to help himself when a gradient of adverse environmental and organizational conditions prevails. Self-help implies both access to health information and a redistribution of responsibility for health from administrators, politicians and professionals to the people: but this cannot be achieved in any effective and stable way without a corresponding redistribution of social power.

Black: One of the pioneers of occupational health, Thomas Legge, said that safety devices in industry had to be such that the worker could not remove them to get a greater output.

Rogers: I don't altogether agree with Dr Saracci about self-help. If one takes this to the extreme, one can say it is the duty of government to produce the ideal environment in which people may help themselves. This is an impossible task. With all our faults, in the developed countries material conditions, including health care, have improved enormously in the last generation, yet the amount of self-help is almost certainly much less, and the seeking of help from government much more, than ever before. I find this very frightening indeed. I am of the tough school which says that in whatever conditions one starts, one must start with self-help. This is one's primary personal responsibility.

Fliedner: The ten-year programme for 'Research and Technology in the Service of Health', which is being prepared in Germany takes some of the problems you mentioned into consideration, Sir Philip (see pp. 163–165).

References

[1] BLACK, D. A. K. & POLE, J. D. (1975) Priorities in biomedical research: indices of burden. *British Journal of Preventive and Social Medicine 29*, 222-227

[2] LYNCH, M. A. (1975) Ill-health and child abuse. *Lancet 2*, 317-319

[3] ROGHMANN, K. J. & HAGGERTY, R. J. (1973) Daily stress, illness, and use of health services in young families. *Pediatric Research 7*, 520-526

International coordination of biomedical research

S. G. OWEN

Medical Research Council, London

Abstract Recent efforts at international coordination in biomedical research have taken place at two levels. At the level of the working clinician and scientist, European regionalism has become increasingly manifest in such organizations as the European Society for Clinical Investigation, the European Organization for Research into the Treatment of Cancer, the European Molecular Biology Organization and many others. These have developed largely, though not entirely, independently of government funding. At the level of science policy, i.e. of bodies supporting biomedical research mainly from public funds, the major developments have been the Comité de la Recherche Médicale of the European Community and the much wider association of European Medical Research Councils, based on the whole of Western Europe; in October 1975 the latter group became incorporated into the new European Science Foundation as the first Standing Committee of that body. Wider, interregional, cooperation presents greater problems, though there have been some modest successes, and the multinational drive on research into six of the major health problems of the third world now being proposed by WHO holds further promise for the future.

The search for an effective western European dimension has dominated efforts at international coordination in biomedical research as seen from the UK during the last three or four years. It seems appropriate to initiate a discussion on international coordination in medical science by briefly reviewing recent and current developments in this part of the world.

Medical research has of course always transcended national boundaries. From the Middle Ages, the growth of medical knowledge has depended on communication and collaboration within the Western World, first the old world, and more latterly within the great anglophone scientific community formed by the addition of the new. The recent renaissance of regionalism has occurred broadly at two levels. One of these is the level at which it has always existed, that of the working scientist and clinician, the laboratory bench and the ward bedside. Here the new Europeanism has become increasingly manifest in the formation of such organizations as the European Society for Clinical Investigation, the European Molecular Biology Organization, the European Training Programme in Brain and Behaviour Research, the European Organization for Research into the Treatment of Cancer and many others. These have developed largely though not entirely independently of government funding, and the activities of some have run much wider than those of ordinary scientific societies. For example, the general programme of the European Molecular Biology Organization (EMBO) comprises short-term and long-term visiting fellowships, professorial fellowships, summer schools and workshops in addition to scientific meetings; the excellence and the effectiveness of this programme are well known, and it has made an important contribution to the creation of a European community in the biological sciences. Since 1970 EMBO has been supported by an intergovernmental financial agreement to which fourteen western European states together with Israel subscribe. The European Training Programme in Brain and Behaviour Research (ETPBBR) is developing along similar lines, and this is also being supported by official funds.

The other level at which European coordination is beginning to occur, and this is an entirely new phenomenon, is that of science policy. By this I mean coordination and collaboration between national organizations responsible for the support of biomedical research mainly or exclusively from public funds. Two major developments have occurred here, one within and one outside the framework of the Common Market. These are the formation of the Comité de la Recherche Médicale (CRM) of the European Community, and the formation of the European Medical Research Council group (EMRC), now incorporated with the new European Science Foundation (ESF). Though both have developed within the context of political and economic changes in western Europe, both are sustained by the growing realization that it is no longer sensible to take far-reaching priority decisions in national isolation. In virtually all the countries concerned, public funds available for the support of biomedical research have ceased to enjoy the generous annual growth rate characteristic of the 1950s and 1960s and are now asymptotic to a constant proportion of gross national product; the most optimistic estimate for the foreseeable future is that the proportion will remain constant, and in the event it may well prove to decline. Against this background and that of the ever-increasing costs and sophistication of scientific research, the need for multinational consultation and cooperation is clear even though the development of common policies must inevitably mean some reordering of national priorities and some sacrifice of national independence in research policy.

The Comité de la Recherche Médicale is the Medical Research Committee of the European Economic Community. It was created in October 1972 as a subcommittee of the Scientific and Technical Research Committee (CREST), through which it reports to the Council of Ministers. It began by organizing training programmes and seminars within the Common Market countries, and is now concentrating on specific and active collaborative projects in relation to traffic accidents, to monitoring of the seriously ill, and to deafness. The Committee has made it a point of principle to operate through national organizations, planning and coordinating activities from Brussels rather than financing research directly from central funds.

Outside the framework of the Community, a number of western European medical research councils or equivalent organizations have been endeavouring to cooperate with each other since 1971, when a Scandinavian initiative brought the executive heads of ten such bodies together in Copenhagen. The original group (Belgium, Denmark, France, Federal Republic of Germany, Ireland, Italy, The Netherlands, Norway, Sweden and the United Kingdom), now enlarged by the addition of Finland, Switzerland and Austria, have continued to meet at regular six-monthly intervals since that time. The attendance of the Director of the US National Institutes of Health as an observer has provided a link with the wider international scene in biomedical research and helped to guard against European parochialism. The primary function of the European Medical Research Council group has been communication, and a regular feature of their meetings is the exchange of information about current scientific policies. The results of particular scientific review studies carried out in one country are circulated to all other members. More active initiatives have been taken where these have seemed appropriate; the group has for example an active subcommittee on toxicology working in a European context. Another subcommittee is examining the financial problems now faced by European medical journals, with the objective of developing common policies towards such questions as page charges and financial subsidies; and the EMRC has concerned itself with a number of other such matters of mutual interest, including multinational clinical trials.

In October 1975 the EMRC group was subsumed into the European Science Foundation, which constitutes the outstanding new development in European scientific collaboration. The formation of such a foundation embracing the whole of fundamental scientific enquiry was first mooted in June 1972 by Signor Spinelli, the then Commissioner of the European Community for Science and Technology, in proposals he put to the Council of Ministers for a common EEC policy in scientific research and technological development. The idea was received by scientists at the non-governmental level with some reservation.

The Royal Society and the Max-Planck Gesellschaft convened meetings in 1972 and 1973 at which doubts were expressed about using the EEC as a template for a scientific organization. The natural unit for scientific cooperation was felt rather to be the whole of western Europe; and it was further considered that joint action by the academics and research councils was preferable to a formal intergovernmental organization. However, to avoid the possibility of having two rival bodies, the idea of a link with the European Community was borne in mind and successive commissioners (Dahrendorf, Brunner) cooperated in subsequent developments, the orginal Spinelli proposals being dropped. After much preparatory work, the new-style ESF finally emerged in October 1974 as an international non-governmental association of organizations 'devoted to the promotion of basic research, its scope including equally the humanities, jurisprudence, social sciences, economics, natural, medical and technical sciences'. Since we are meeting under the auspices of the Ciba Foundation, it is appropriate that at this point I should recall the important part played in the creation of the ESF by Professor Hubert Bloch, Founder's representative on the Executive Council of the Ciba Foundation from 1968 until his death in May 1974. Bloch was an active member of the ESF Preparatory Commission, and it was the 'Bloch formula' which neatly solved the sensitive problem of how to allocate voting rights to national groups of organizations. Tragically, he died before the ESF was finally and formally established.

Organizations eligible to become members of the ESF are national bodies in European countries which support basic research 'from significant means assigned for that purpose' by the government of the country. Founder members were drawn from sixteen countries: Austria, Belgium, Denmark, France, Germany, Greece, Ireland, Italy, The Netherlands, Norway, Portugal, Spain, Sweden, Switzerland, United Kingdom and Yugoslavia. The largest national group of members is that of the UK, which has seven: the Royal Society, the British Academy and the five Research Councils (Science, Social Science, Medical, Agricultural and Natural Environment). In all, forty-three academies and research councils now adhere to the ESF. It seems possible that the ideal of a single European research council may be in sight and that further prolifer-ation of separate agreements and treaties such as that referred to in relation to molecular biology will be unnecessary. Already, for example, the European Training Programme in Brain and Behaviour Research is under consideration for support as an 'additional activity' of the ESF, and other initiatives on bio-medical research are certain to follow.

I hope that this distinguished international group will not think me unduly parochial in illustrating the topic of international coordination in biomedical research by reviewing western European regional developments. Wider interregional cooperation presents greater problems, but before concluding I should like to mention the plans now being formulated by a number of national and international aid agencies, under the leadership of the United Nations Development Programme and WHO, for a concerted attack on research into the major health problems of the Third World, notably into malaria, schistosomiasis, filariasis, trypanosomiasis, leprosy and leishmaniasis. At the moment, these plans are only on paper, but if they are even partly successful, they will constitute a milestone in the development of international collaborative medical research.

I should like to end by re-emphasizing a point I made earlier, namely that international coordination of biomedical research must necessarily involve a degree of sacrifice of independent national research policy on the part of collaborating organizations and nations. My view is that this has been insufficiently recognized and, so far, certainly insufficiently achieved.

Discussion

Fliedner: The basis for scientific cooperation is the same at the national as at the international level. It is also the same for the bench worker as for large organizations. That basis is what I call the three Cs: competence, creativity and confidence.[1] These three elements are vital, and they lead to cooperation through what we call the club stage. Clearly, there can be no scientific cooperation unless the participants, individuals as well as organizations, are extremely competent. And without creativity there would be no progress. In international as well as national terms, confidence in each other is of the highest importance. Scientific cooperation at all levels is impaired when the partners do not have enough confidence in each other to work together.

The question has been raised (p. 69) of how one gets cooperation or collaboration, and it was suggested that clubs have to be formed first, a club being defined as an informal gathering of friends who learn to work with each other and talk to each other. I have seen several attempts at international collaboration fail when this club stage of development was not carefully pursued. An example of success is the EORTC Gnotobiotic Project Group. The EORTC organizes clinical cooperative trials, one of which deals with whether patients with leukaemia benefit from being treated in a sterile environment under sterile conditions. It took this group about two years of the club stage to become an effectively cooperating group, and it is now preparing its first publication on a prospective randomized study in Europe. I think it takes that long before competent and creative people have enough confidence in each other to work together. This confidence has to extend to the sensitive point of priority in publication. Only among friends can one say something that in principle could be exploited by somebody else. This type of confidence is very important because when we talk to each other as scientists in the basic sciences we are holding out signed cheques which could be cashed by anybody who took them away.

Confidence becomes important between organizations too. In Europe many of our organizations have not yet worked together enough. I am glad that the European Medical Research Council representatives have now had about three years of the club stage, working on some interesting problems. The club stage is usually occupied with something non-committal, such as standardization of methods, during which people learn whether they can agree with each other.

In Europe one problem is that there is no organization to which cooperative groups can apply for what we call 'catalytic money'. Catalytic money is needed when people in different places want to work together in a coherent system. They need catalytic money for the essential club meetings, for secretarial work, postage and publication, and so on. I and other people have written letters to the European Medical Research Council representatives and to the European Science Foundation but have never had a positive response. Administrators are of course very suspicious when people ask for money for meetings. That is not usually considered to be an appropriate way of spending public funds. But for creating true collaboration and coordination meetings are essential; written communications are not enough. Perhaps in twenty years from now short-circuit television will eliminate the need for physical meeting, but television costs even more than air fares.

Here I should say a word of gratitude to both the Ciba Foundation and the Wellcome Trust. These two organizations have seen the necessity for catalytic expenditure and have provided funds for this type of thing, the Wellcome Trust by promoting bilateral research arrangements between countries, and the Ciba Foundation by holding symposia and in various other ways. But public funds are also needed for this purpose.

In 1961 when the European Economic Community was coming into being, an American asked whether the creation of the EEC should be considered as a threat or as something positive. At that time one of our American colleagues wrote 'We must have the European Community because we need a competent partner in this world'. I think this is true, and we have failed so far to form this scientific partnership, a partnership which is essential in a world where Europe is in the process of being crushed between big power blocs that will eventually also turn out to be big scientific powers.

Meyer: I do not completely share your somewhat pessimistic attitude, Dr

Fliedner. Since the first meeting of the European Society for Clinical Investigation in 1966 I have felt that cooperation in clinical investigation in Europe has been excellent. The efforts of the Ciba Foundation, the Wellcome Trust and other bodies in various European countries have helped to achieve considerable progress. I agree however that some things could be improved, such as the availability of catalytic money.

Dr Owen said that some sacrifice would be needed by European countries wishing to achieve their scientific goals, and the hypertension trial provides an example. I think that this trial is necessary, although it may not bring the results we expect or solve all the problems. On the other hand it is very expensive and it seems wrong that Great Britain alone in Europe, should suffer from this. I am also aware that the medical structure in the UK helps to make medical trials much better than in any other country in Europe. The non-British European countries should in this matter accept that the trial is necessary and that it should be held in England, and that therefore they should agree to pay for it. This implies a sacrifice, of course. I therefore wonder whether the decision of the European Science Foundation to be a non-intergovernmental organization is wise. We are still dealing with a complex political situation, and interaction should perhaps start between politicians and scientists.

Owen: The word 'non-intergovernmental' is perhaps misleading. Almost all the member organizations require the approval of their governments to engage in international activity. In fact governments play quite a large part. The European Science Foundation was made a non-intergovernmental organization to avoid the cumbersome necessity of having an international treaty which would take a long time to be approved by every country.

Burgen: The European Training Programme in Brain and Behaviour Research (ETPBBR) was originally set up because it was felt that neurosciences research in Europe was lagging behind that in North America, largely because it was fragmented. The whole philosophy of the organization was that it should have exactly the catalytic role that Dr Fliedner referred to and use its money in the catalytic role, setting up arrangements between laboratories whose abilities in, say, behavioural research and neurophysiological research complement each other. There is money for travel and subsistence, and for sending people for training to various places. In other words there is a club. They organize interdisciplinary conferences, and hold a regular winter school in Switzerland on various aspects of neuroscience. The catalytic role has been immensely successful. This programme really became active in 1970 and in this five-year trial period there has been a perceptible improvement in the quality of research and in the development of interdisciplinary areas of research, which in the nervous system are especially important. It is encouraging that this has been done with government money.

Owen: The ESF has so far been cautious about providing catalytic money. Its statutes allow it to use funds this way, and there is a mechanism whereby member organizations need subscribe to such activities only if they wish to do so. Two organizations, the ETPBBR and the IHES (the Institute for Higher Scientific Studies at Bur-sur-Yvette), are supported by member organizations of the ESF but not within the framework of the ESF. I hope that the ESF will cut its teeth on these two and will then go on to all the others.

Fliedner: I want to encourage you to help the European Science Foundation to get its feet wet in this way, Dr Owen. It should not consider that clinical research and clinical trial research are too far removed from science to be its concern.

Saracci: Health services research, at least on paper, offers plenty of opportunity for cooperation within Europe. There are enough similarities and enough differences between the health services and the local conditions, and a lot could be done. The communication channels in health services research are not as good as in clinical investigation, for example, and we should try to find a mechanism for catalysing communication at this level.

Dr Fliedner's remarks about competence and creativity are very relevant. In Italy there are at present very few competent people in the prospective field of health services research. Within the framework of CRM there are a number of groups, one of which is the Specialized Working Group on Epidemiological and Statistical Research and Clinical Trials. This EEC group is trying to bring together people who are by training concerned with problems in epidemiology, including health services research. Health services research is also a prominent concern of a non-governmental group, the Panel for Social Medicine and Epidemiology in the European Community, which represents research workers and epidemiology associations in the EEC countries and whose beginnings were catalysed by the Ciba Foundation. These are good initiatives, but one must acknowledge that there is still a large discrepancy between the potential opportunities in health services research and what is actually done, especially in continental Europe.

Luft: Some years ago I was asked by the Swedish government to set up a health care programme for diabetes; after about two years I got interested in this and drew up a scheme. In the meantime, as President of the International Diabetes Federation, I had looked at health care programmes for diabetic patients in other countries and found that no country had found a useful programme. The programme that I thought would be suitable for Sweden is now being discussed there. I had found that about the same health care programme could also be used in the Sudan, South Africa, Egypt, Israel, and Cuba. My programme is now being tried in different countries, and this is a sort of international collaboration. In Cuba they have tried it for two years and it works beautifully. But resistance in a highly developed country like Sweden is tough.

In developing countries—such as the Sudan—I was invariably asked whether something could be done for diabetic research. The health care programme is all right: it costs money but it will eventually save money, but they feel they must start research because otherwise they can't get the doctors interested. It is difficult to start research in some countries, but it is possible. For example, there is a big island in Khartoum where the people, although quite well off, intermarry a hundred per cent. It happened that a Dean of the Medical School came from that tribe. This inbred strain of people should be a beautiful starting point for looking for prediabetes, latent diabetes and so on. In simple ways like that we can start research on an international basis.

Reference

[1] FLIEDNER, T. M. (1976): Three 'C': A Challenge. (Presidential Address 1975 of the European Society for Clinical Investigation). *European Journal of Clinical Investigation 6*, 1-5

General discussion:
Research, practice and education

Black: At this symposium we have been hearing about the nature of medical practice and about various forms of research. The two areas of course interact and overlap. We should now consider whether, in research, there is any justification for a hierarchy based on levels of biological organization from the molecule up through the organelle, the cell, the tissue, the system, the organism, and the society. Another question is the feasibility of introducing the concept of social responsibility into the 'direction' of research. And we have already talked a lot about the importance of health services research, its feasibility and the status it enjoys (pp. 151–167).

The most important thing to consider, however, is probably the first point, the interaction between research and practice. Clearly, both of these are fairly complex activities and we would be optimistic if we expected to find many one-to-one relationships between them. But they have some common ground. Ideally a critical and objective approach should underlie both. In medical practice, of course, there is something called empathy that is difficult to define and which is often more tolerant than critical. Similarly, in research it is easy to underestimate the emotional involvement of the research worker. Polanyi[1] gives many telling examples of this. We might also ask: should a research outlook inform both practice and teaching? To me that is merely a rhetorical question: teaching and practice will both wither away unless people have the kind of approach which informs good research. Conversely, and this is a much more difficult question, how far should perceived problems of practice influence the direction of the research effort?

Eisenberg: The clinical trial of anti-hypertensive drugs provoked a good deal of controversy during this meeting. It is sadly true that the information gathered at great expense by such efforts rarely feeds back into practice. We should perhaps stipulate that the design of the research should include a set of pro-

207

positions about how the information will get back into the practice of physicians. One way to do that is to involve the physicians themselves in the process of obtaining the information. A potential virtue of the British scheme for developing facilities for general practititoners is that information retrieval systems could make it possible for the doctor to discover which of the things he has done has benefited the patients most. The more involved the doctor is in this process —the more he is oriented towards looking for information—perhaps the more likely he is to be a consumer of that information.

Involving the doctor in securing information will lead him to modify his behaviour, because then he will be getting information from which he benefits either economically or in delivering health care. When one does things that seem to work but never finds out whether they really work, one routinely goes on doing them. How do we get the information in the first place? The trial of anti-hypertensive agents is likely to tell us whether they are effective. Once we have that information, what will make doctors change their prescribing behaviour if the differences are statistically significant only when very large populations are examined? It is really the cigarette smoking and lung cancer problem: if people dropped dead after the first cigarette, or even the tenth, no one would smoke, but it takes a whole lot of cigarettes, and only some of the people who smoke die. We need intermediate feedback to change behaviour.

Dollery: One of the reasons why therapeutic trials have not been well developed in some countries is that in independent systems of practice it is difficult to do such simple things as to control the patients in the trial. It is certainly much easier for us to do the hypertension trial in the UK than it would be in most other countries in Europe.

In independent systems it is also more difficult to implement the results of health care research, because access to the practitioners is limited. In fact it is also limited in the UK because the general practitioners have kept their independent contractor status even within the reorganized National Health Service. Although I sympathize with what has been said about undergraduate education, I do not think that that is the long-term answer, nor is postgraduate education. Even in the UK, where there is a positive financial incentive for general practitioners to attend postgraduate instruction, two-thirds of them scarcely bother. Anyway, lectures by visiting firemen, which is what this kind of instruction consists of, has little impact. What we need is an audit system. Within a hospital, peer pressure is a form of audit, but this is lacking in general practice, although attempts are being made to organize it. But the general practitioners' lack of knowledge is not an argument for not doing things like the hypertension trial: we must have evidence that one way of doing things is better than another.

Marinker: I agree. We have been using the word 'research' in a number of different senses, one of which refers simply to the training it provides in scientific method. This is important in making doctors aware of what they are doing and of its effects. This kind of education can, I believe, change people's behaviour, but the education of primary care doctors has gone wrong because, as Dr Dollery said, it has consisted of lectures which, however erudite, do not seem relevant to the practitioner. We must look at research as a tool of education. That is, audit must become the main educational method for doctors outside hospitals as well as inside them.

Pickering: The research problems seem to divide themselves into two broad categories, one biomedical, including the hard sciences, and the other socio-medical. In both these categories the only effective way of answering questions is by interdisciplinary collaboration. This has always mattered in my own work on hypertension because the problems could not be solved inside my own department of medicine. It seemed better to try to collaborate with other people who really knew their subject than for me to try to learn their techniques and then do the work rather badly. The people with whom I was able to work had open minds, they listened and got interested in new problems. One of Wilfred Trotter's best sayings was that the most powerful antigen known to man is a new idea. Certainly, most people faced with a new idea instantly reject it and the people with whom one can work are the people who are prepared to let a new idea enter into their minds and see how it works out.

Another problem is language, not foreign languages but the technological jargon that every discipline wraps around itself as a sort of camouflage or defence. We doctors are terribly bad about this but the sociologists are perhaps worse. I think this is the chief barrier to collaboration between doctors and social scientists.

An important point about education, mentioned already (p. 69; p. 193) is the desirability of students moving out of their own narrow disciplines and into others. But this is getting progressively more difficult, especially for medical students. In one school which thinks itself very progressive they have sixty examinations in the first two years; this is called continuous assessment but it is really discontinuous examination. The students complain that they are constantly glued to the lecture theatre and their books, and never have time to get interested in anything else. This is terribly dangerous to the future of collaborative research.

Woodruff: Research in clinical departments seems to fall into three distinct categories: research as pure occupational therapy for the people doing it, research as part of the teaching function, and research which is really intended to discover new things. This last kind seems impossible to achieve in a clinical department without interdisciplinary collaboration, and there are two ways of trying to get that collaboration. One is to persuade colleagues in other departments to get involved, which is often extremely difficult. The other way is to attract scientists of quality in their own discipline to work in clinical departments. We have always had two or three such people in the Department of Surgery in Edinburgh, and they have been enormously helpful in eliminating the element of amateurishness which characterizes a good deal of clinical research. For their part, they have found that the feedback from clinical practice has generated ideas that have formed interesting starting points for basic research. I think that this sort of partnership should be developed on a much bigger scale. It is becoming increasingly difficult to maintain such arrangements however, because, faced with a financial crisis, the University begins to question the function of these scientists in relation to what it regards as the main task of the Department, which is teaching medical students. As the answer is 'very little', the scientists are liable, in present conditions, to be the first to be axed. But if university clinical departments have an important function in contributing to new discoveries, as I think they have, the part played by the basic scientists is essential, and it would be a pity to lose them.

Berliner: In our experience at Yale it has been difficult to obtain good basic scientists for clinical departments, not because they are likely to get the axe but because they can't see a real future for themselves in those departments and they tend to be looked down upon by colleagues from their own disciplinary departments. It is much better for them to have a primary appointment in their own discipline, with a secondary appointment and possibly even housing in another department.

Black: This would apply equally to sociologists, of course.

Hiatt: One way in which that problem has been successfully approached has been to offer education and training in biology to physicians who then go into clinical investigation with backgrounds in both biology and medicine. Those people have also served to improve communications between departments of biological sciences and clinical departments. Now we are faced with the need to bring other disciplines to bear on health problems. For example, how do we encourage experts in other disciplines to think about such complex and important questions as how to get people to stop smoking cigarettes or what we can do to bring about greater effectiveness and efficiency in health services.

These questions are in some ways as complicated and enigmatic as was the structure of haemoglobin thirty years ago. As Dr Dornhorst implied earlier (p. 193), people trained in medicine are not qualified to address these questions without help. How do we encourage the most able scholars from other disciplines to enter very complicated health areas in a way that ensures that they interact with medical people on the one hand, and that they continue their relationships with colleagues in their own disciplines, on the other? At Harvard we are exploring methods of so doing. For example, our Center for the Analysis of Health Practices brings together physicians, economists, statisticians, lawyers, policy analysts, biologists and others, and their students, from throughout the University. Working groups are concerned with such issues as a national policy for hypertension, legal and ethical aspects of experimentation in human subjects, cost–benefit aspects of such surgical procedures as tonsillectomy and hysterectomy, and problems of diffusion of medical technology. Several papers and books have emerged from joint research efforts. The Center is promoting an interest in thorny health problems on the part of distinguished scholars from throughout Harvard and may be serving to interest students from several disciplines in health careers. Finally, it is demonstrating to most of us the substantial obstacles to, but the far more substantial gratifications from, interdisciplinary health research.

Fliedner: I am an active participant in an experiment that may provide some answers to the problem of how to attract the best people to the medical schools. The German government thought that the new medical faculty at Ulm should be a simple medical school, educating only medical students, but the founding committee persuaded the government to accept something different. We said that we would not be able to attract the best physicists, chemists, biologists or mathematicians to teach first and second-year students in a medical school unless those teachers had the incentive of being able to train students in their own disciplines. So what we created was a School of Science and Medicine. The architects had to find a way of bringing medicine and natural sciences close together, essentially under one roof, to encourage interdisciplinary thinking and activity. In this scheme the clinical centre, with departments of internal medicine, surgery and neurosciences, is linked to biology, theoretical medicine, physics, chemistry and mathematics by what we call the 'centre of basic clinical research'. Our feeling was that professionals who understand both the clinical and the basic scientific language are needed to catalyse the interaction between biology etc. and the clinical centre. (By language I mean the methodological language which enables those people to translate clinical problems into experimental approaches.) The decisive point is that everyone is in one building so that it will be easy to go from any place in the building to the bedside and back to the laboratory. Even in the short time since 1967 there has been plenty of collaboration between physics, biology and medicine.

At the very beginning we also asked what, in hard-core physics, is relevant to biology and medicine, and what, in clinical problems, requires hard-core physics to be done. So most of the people we first appointed to chairs were working in molecular structural research, which is an important part of physical chemistry. Even though about 80% of the human body consists of water, very little is known about the structure of water, and problems in physics and chemistry are clearly extremely relevant to the understanding of biological problems.

Randle: In 1969 the clinical research centre at the Université de Montreal had a laboratory block with a director who not only ran his own research programme but also provided laboratory facilities for other clinical departments. I wonder how that particular experiment has worked out?

In the UK an unprecedented amount of money has been spent in the last fifteen years on refurbishing universities and increasing their accommodation, yet large new teaching hospitals have been built with very little laboratory accommodation. Moreover, the basic sciences which could have serviced medicine have been segregated in totally different buildings. I cannot understand why we cannot build science departments in university hospitals and let them do their science there, on the pattern Dr Fliedner has just described.

Dr Fliedner also implied that if we want collaboration, there have to be people willing to form the links. If the body wants catalysis it makes catalysts; if it wants to concentrate efforts it puts handles on molecules so that they become attached to a common surface at an appropriate moment. Similarly, if we want to improve interfaces, we must create individuals who will make the links. One of the weak points of all categories of medical research is that we haven't solved the problems of identifying individuals who are good at this sort of thing or of providing them with career opportunities. I am not convinced by the argument that these people have no educational role. After all, if there is one first-class biochemist in a hospital who over twenty years has educated the physicians in that hospital, he has fulfilled as important a role as if he had an influence on three or four hundred undergraduates.

Campbell: At McMaster University the architecture of the medical school has a similar objective to that Dr Fliedner described for Ulm. We also tried tackling the problem of how to preserve the biochemist in his intellectual home while he cooperates with members of other departments on problems of shared interest. We have created a physical and organizational medium which I hope will be extremely liberal in its educational influence, but there are pressures, both from the students and from the teachers, which tend to create a pressure-cooker medical school rather than an educational environment.

Hjort: We must remember that every scheme has unintentional side effects. Dr Meyer (pp. 137–145) gave us the example of INSERM which was designed to produce the very best for medicine, but unintentionally turned out rather differently. If European collaborative research is going to be in huge institutions far away from the front line, it will do science more good than it does medicine. The public may rescue the professionals from this kind of mistake, because the public may in many instances have a better overall view. It is important for us to make room for public influence, both in research and in practice. But if the public is to have more influence, it also needs more education, and we ourselves must supply that education, which raises difficult issues.

Dornhorst: How can we steer worth-while research in directions which central bodies consider desirable? From my experience at the MRC, I don't think we know at all how do do this.

Black: I certainly don't know the answer to that. One might imagine that any thoughtful clinician should know what is important and what is not, but that simple starting point has been undermined by sociologists, epidemiologists and many others. I don't think we can ever really escape value judgements, which in theory ought to be made by the public, but by whom among the public? If we say it is the representatives we have elected to parliament then I am not sure that this is self-evidently a better decision-making system than the professional decision-making system we have been using.

At this meeting I have been impressed particularly by the need for interdisciplinary collaboration. This is certainly one of the things which is going to be cardinal to future progress. While monodisciplinary activity solves many problems at a tactical level, I think that at the strategic level one has to have multidisciplinary activity. The contribution of the Ciba Foundation in bringing such a diverse group together at this meeting is a practical example of what can be done.

References

[1] POLANYI, M. (1956) Passion and controversy in science. *Lancet 1*, 921-925

Index of contributors

Entries in **bold** type indicate papers; other entries refer to discussion contributions

Indexes compiled by William Hill

Subject index